# Advocacy

# Acclaim for
# NCPed's Advocacy

"**Dave Tayloe and his co-authors** have created a deeply moving and hugely practical account of the dedication and long-term commitment of scores of people in North Carolina who have collaborated to build a comprehensive and responsive health care system for children in their state. The story is told by an impressive group of clinicians, health care managers, academics, and policy-makers, as well as leaders of the North Carolina Chapter of the American Academy of Pediatrics."

   *Judith S. Palfrey, MD, FAAP*

"**This book gives a great mix of the broad strokes,** infrastructure, and focus on how North Carolina health professionals did what was best for children and families. The book is sprinkled with individual stories from many of the actual players, telling in detail how things happened. The enthusiasm and commitment shine through, along with the way the advocacy work changed them as people, awakening leadership skills some did not know they had. Yet, throughout the different stories, a theme continues to emerge: relationships count! Success as an advocate or advocacy organization is hugely dependent on finding common ground with collaborators and strengthening the relationships over time. The book is rich with examples of how the pediatricians and their partners improved the well-being and health of North Carolina children and families."

   *Renée R. Jenkins, MD, FAAP*

# Fifty Years of Advocacy

## THE NORTH CAROLINA PEDIATRIC SOCIETY

**ISBN 979-8-218-24998-4 (PBK)**

First edition 2023

Edited by Dave Tayloe Jr., MD, FAAP
Associate Editor Steve Shore, MSW
Copyedited by Lara Hammer Ivanitch, Paige Hachet Jacob, and Neosha Hough Smith
Book design by Kristin Erb, Blend Media Boutique

Printed in the United States of America by
Versa Press, Inc., 1465 Spring Bay Road, East Peoria, IL 61611.

Published by Grateful Steps Foundation, Crest Mountain,
30 Ben Lippen School Road #107, Asheville, NC 28806.
www.gratefulsteps.org

To everyone who sees
the wonder in children
and works tirelessly to assure that
all children have a body that is healthy and well
and a mind that is alive with curiosity
and a spirit blessed with
a future of hope and excitement.

# Table of Contents

## APPENDIX

# Foreword

## Lessons Learned from the North Carolina Pediatric Society

Since its inception in 1930, the American Academy of Pediatrics (AAP) has advocated for the health and welfare of children, both in the clinical setting and within the larger community, to effect systemic change. In the 1980s, there was a return to federalism, in which the Reagan and Bush administrations delegated more authority to the states to address children's health policy rather than imposing federal mandates. AAP chapters had new opportunities to enhance children's health coverage through Medicaid expansions, but had to convince state governments to accept the federal matching funds. Although chapters were and remain independent entities, the AAP administration invested in a "State Advocacy Coordinator" to help state chapters mount their advocacy campaigns. I began in that role in May of 1986.

Getting to know the leaders of the fifty-nine AAP chapters consisted of multiple phone calls and meetings during the chapter chairman's forum (there were only three women presidents in 1986) as the commercial internet was not yet available. I quickly began to assess which chapters had legislative experience, which were successful, which had established meaningful connections, and which had leaders who could serve as mentors for other chapters. North Carolina was among a small cadre of chapters that had a system in place to successfully advocate for children's health policy.

During the spring of 1988, the AAP convened its first legislative conference in Washington, DC, and Dave Tayloe Jr. was invited to discuss the vaccine liability bill that created the vaccine injury compensation program the North Carolina Legislature had enacted in 1986 to stem the tide of litigation related to the pertussis vaccine. The North Carolina state law preceded the National Vaccine Program and compensation program later the same year. I was the one who called Dr. Tayloe to ask if he would be willing to speak at the inaugural legislative conference. So began our working relationship of more than thirty-five years.

As I learned many years ago and as presented in this book, the North Carolina Chapter had developed an infrastructure to support their child advocacy work. The relationships and accompanying communication between the North Carolina Pediatric Society, state government officials, and the four medical schools in the state constituted a powerful force to design and implement policy that promoted children's health and welfare. The liaison committee meetings (later called open forum meetings) were a key component of the North Carolina Pediatric Society's advocacy success. Trusted relationships, ongoing communication, and a vested interest in improving children's health and well-being were the ingredients of effective advocacy and the resulting successful policy. The AAP promoted the concept of open forum meetings to other AAP Chapters through Chapter communications and District meetings.

In this volume you will discover how this "formula" was applied to numerous issues over the years with the same successful results. Focusing on children's needs rather than institutional or individual needs was key, whether the policy in question was health insurance coverage, child abuse prevention, newborn screening, or mental health services. Children's needs always came first; data and accountability were key and adequate payment to the providers was part of the system to assure the services could be delivered in a timely fashion.

Participation by the provider community was seen as assuring the delivery system was in place. Leadership also was a key component to NCPeds. There seemed to be an abundance of talented pediatric leaders in the state, as you will read in this book. Yet in reality, they learned from each other and mentored the younger members to be able to step into leadership roles, another key component to the NCPeds' advocacy success.

– *Judith C. Dolins, MPH*
*Former Chief Implementation Officer and Senior Vice President, Community and Chapter Affairs and Quality Improvement, American Academy of Pediatrics*

# Preface

## Introduction and Purpose

**by the NCPeds Steering Committee**

This book should be of value to all health professionals who understand that we will only have an optimal, functional health care system if frontline health professionals are involved and play a leading role in designing and implementing the holistic system of care. For the past fifty years, the NC Pediatric Society/NC Chapter of the American Academy of Pediatrics (NCPeds) has worked with state government leaders and administrators, private sector health and human service entities, and other like-minded advocacy groups to design and implement a child health system that assures that all providers of child health services can afford to offer all children access to comprehensive health services in a medical home.

This publication is an attempt by former and current leaders of NCPeds to explain how and why one state's provider organization developed the administrative infrastructure necessary to support frontline health professionals in their efforts to significantly improve the system of care for children. Two documents were extremely helpful to the NCPeds Steering Committee in developing the text. These include "A History of the North Carolina Pediatric Society and the North Carolina Chapter of the American Academy of Pediatrics," by Peter English, MD, PhD (1982), and "A History of the North Carolina Pediatric Society from 1980-2014" (2015) by Steve Shore, MSW.

Our publication describes some of the many advocacy efforts of NCPeds during the past fifty years. The commentaries are the reflections of many of the key leaders and influencers across the past five decades of NCPeds' history. The commentaries reveal important truths about the passion and "smarts" pediatricians bring to advocating for child health, the importance of infrastructure, and the effectiveness and fun of having many dance partners at the advocacy party.

Advocacy for children, families, and pediatricians is the primary focus of the American Academy of Pediatrics (AAP) State Chapters. The North Carolina Chapter of the AAP does not pretend to have all the secrets to successful advocacy, but we have rich infrastructure traditions that have allowed us to implement many successful advocacy campaigns throughout the organization's history.

Our purpose is to demonstrate how a dedicated small organization can make a dramatic difference in opportunities for children. Our hope is that others will be inspired to enhance their own advocacy efforts. Children are our future—we must assertively ensure a fertile environment for their growth and development.

We believe that successful advocacy requires the following elements:

- An open forum, continuing education programs, and effective communication methods. These raise awareness of issues that must be addressed to improve the health and safety of children, identify those issues that require system-level interventions, and foster dialog among our members and other stakeholders (individuals and groups affected by the issues), as well as government officials about root causes and potential systemic solutions.
- Collaboration with key stakeholders, typically through meeting together. This type of combined efforts tap into members' and stakeholders' expertise and experience in addressing the issues; develop a full range of strategies to address the identified issues such as need for additional resources, enhanced clinical and business practices, educational initiatives (public and professional), engagement of additional partners, and policy changes (changes in school or agency rules and procedures, state or local legislation, appropriations); and achieve consensus among key stakeholders as to prioritize action steps and persons or groups who could help us implement our advocacy agenda.
- Relationships with local and state agency officials and elected leaders. Fostering these bonds helps forge agreement about needed changes to policies and payment; pursue initiatives that are feasible in the current political environment through the activation of grassroots constituencies, including local pediatricians and parents; and celebrate successes and credit champions and partners.

We hope that readers of this document reflect upon their own experiences advocating for health system improvements, gain insight from our commentaries, and become more successful in their efforts to improve access and quality of care for *all* people.

# Acknowledgments

## NCPeds Steering Committee for Fifty Years of Advocacy: The North Carolina Pediatric Society

**KATHLEEN CLARKE-PEARSON, MD, FAAP**

**Steering Committee Coordinator of Communications**
**Steering Committee Chairperson**

Dr. Clarke-Pearson is a retired general pediatrician and former elementary school teacher who remains very active in child advocacy work both in NC and in the US Congress. She served on the AAP Council on Communications and Media Committee and Executive Committee for many years and is a dedicated mediatrician/tweetiatrician. Dr. Clarke-Pearson also spent six years on the Committee for Federal Government Affairs, meeting several times a year with legislative staffers from our NC Congressional delegation to advocate for CHIP expansion, SNAP reform, and sensible gun violence prevention policies. In February 2021, she and Dr. Tayloe Jr. conceived the idea of a book that would be dedicated to telling the spectacular stories of NC pediatric child advocacy over the last fifty years through our unique and supportive NCPeds. Dr. Clarke-Pearson and her spouse of fifty-one years raised their four children in Chapel Hill and now spend most of their time at their Blue Ridge Mountain Ashe County home. Their three grandchildren live close by. She remains very engaged in raising their three grandchildren to be the future advocates for the environment.

**E. STEPHEN EDWARDS, MD, FAAP**

Dr. Edwards is a co-founder of Raleigh Children and Adolescent Medicine, where he provided general pediatric care for thirty-three years, and served as clinical professor of pediatrics at the University of North Carolina Medical School Department of Pediatrics. His education includes a BS degree from Davidson College, an MD from Duke University Medical School, pediatric education at Emory University, and two years in the US Air Force. His interest in child advocacy drew him to NCPeds where he served multiple positions, including chair of governmental programs, member of the executive committee, vice president, and president. Active in the American Academy of Pediatrics (AAP), he served on the Council on Pediatric Practice, Council

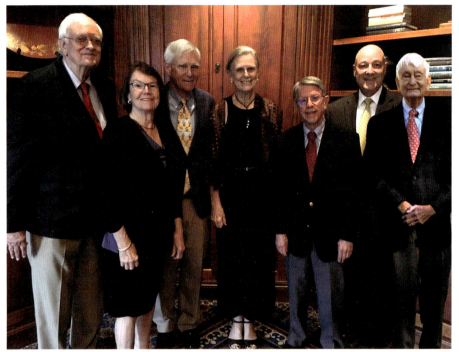

Left to Right: Steve Edwards, Kathleen Clarke-Pearson, Dave Tayloe Jr., Jane Meschan Foy, Bob Schwartz, Steve Shore, Olson Huff

on Government Affairs (chair), District IV vice chair, District IV chair, AAP Board of Directors, president-elect, president, chair of the Sub-Committee on Access, and the Council of Past Presidents (chair). Now retired, he is a Life Master in bridge, plays golf, and continues a forty-six-year low-stakes poker game. He and his wife Sylvia live at The Cypress, a Raleigh retirement community.

## JANE MESCHAN FOY, MD, FAAP

Dr. Foy spent more than forty years practicing pediatrics in primary care, public health, school, and academic settings, most recently as professor of pediatrics at Wake Forest University School of Medicine. There, in addition to her clinical roles, she developed Wake Forest's first advocacy curriculum for residents; co-founded the School Health Alliance for Forsyth County, which established school-based health care programs in the local public schools; and served as medical director of Northwest Community Care (Medicaid) Network. She was president of NCPeds from 1998-2000, then served in several AAP leadership roles, including chair of the Committee on Psychosocial Aspects of Child and Family Health, chair of the

Task Force on Mental Health, District IV vice chair and chair, and member of the AAP Board of Directors. Her publications include lead authorship of the 2019 AAP policy statement, "Mental Health Competencies for Pediatric Practice." Since retiring to Wake Forest's Emeritus Academy, she has served as associate editor of mental health content for Pediatric Care Online. Dr. Foy received her BA from Wellesley College and her MD from the University of North Carolina at Chapel Hill, then completed her pediatric residency at the University of Virginia, Emory University, and UNC hospitals. She and her husband, Miles Foy, live in Oak Ridge, North Carolina.

## OLSON HUFF, MD, FAAP

Dr. Huff is a retired pediatrician. He is medical director emeritus of the Mission Children's Hospital. His medical degree is from the University of Louisville, and his internship was at Wilford Hall US Air Force (USAF) Hospital in San Antonio, Texas. He is a graduate of the USAF School of Aerospace Medicine and served as a flight surgeon in the Vietnam theater in the early stages of that war. He completed his residency in pediatrics at Charlotte Memorial Hospital (now Atrium Health Charlotte) and practiced pediatrics in Charlotte for fourteen years. After moving to Asheville, he established the Olson Huff Center for Child Development and later became the founding medical director of Mission Children's Hospital. He is a past president of NCPeds and served on a number of committees of the American Academy of Pediatrics. He also served as a commissioner on the NC Health and Wellness Trust Fund and as a panel member on numerous NC Institute of Medicine research and policy projects. In retirement, he continues to consult on issues related to childhood autism. He and his wife Marilyn of fifty-nine years lived for many years in Black Mountain, North Carolina, and now reside in Asheville, North Carolina.

## ROBERT SCHWARTZ, MD, FAAP

Dr. Schwartz is professor emeritus of pediatrics at Wake Forest University School of Medicine in Winston-Salem, North Carolina. He received his bachelor of science and medical degrees from the University of Florida, then completed his residency in pediatrics at Carolinas Medical Center in Charlotte, North Carolina, and a fellowship in pediatric endocrinology and metabolism at Duke University Medical Center. Among Dr. Schwartz's state and national activities, he has served as president of NCPeds, and on the Residency Review Committee for Pediatrics and the Maintenance of Certification in Pediatrics Examination Committee of the American Board of Pediatrics. He received the initial NCPeds Academic Service Award in 2002 and the NC Health and Wellness Trust Fund Leadership Award in Preventive Health in 2005. In 2008, Dr. Schwartz received the Outstanding Achievement Award for childhood obesity prevention and, in 2012, the Honorary Membership Award from

NCPeds. Since retiring from clinical practice in 2011, Dr. Schwartz started and has been co-director of the first school food pantry in Forsyth County, which is now in its tenth year of offering healthy food to needy families with a child at a local elementary school. For the past six years, he also has been helping two Syrian refugee families with access to our complicated health care system. He and his wife Rebecca live in Winston-Salem.

**STEVE SHORE, MSW, ASSOCIATE EDITOR**

Steve Shore is a former executive director of NCPeds. He served fifteen years, from 1999 until his retirement in 2014. During his tenure with NCPeds, the chapter was twice recognized as the Outstanding Very Large Chapter by the American Academy of Pediatrics. NCPeds created a foundation to secure funding for charitable projects in 1999. Shore helped bring grants from national philanthropies, including The Robert Wood Johnson Foundation, The Campaign for Tobacco-Free Kids, and Americans Nonsmokers' Rights Foundation. He helped secure additional grants from more than a dozen North Carolina charitable foundations and secured contracts with multiple state government institutions. A native of North Carolina, Shore's career spans thirty-eight years in health care advocacy and management. He helped start and launch five rural community health centers and was a practice manager for two health centers. He then spent twenty-six years as the head of two statewide health care associations, the NC Community Health Center Association and NCPeds. He earned a baccalaureate degree from Duke University and a master of social work degree from Tulane University. He and his wife, Darlene, live in Apex, North Carolina.

# About the Editor: Dave Tayloe Jr., MD, FAAP

Dave Tayloe Jr., MD, FAAP, former president of the American Academy of Pediatrics, is in active pediatric practice. He founded a solo practice in Goldsboro, North Carolina, in 1977, after completing medical school at the University of North Carolina and pediatric residencies at St. Christopher's Hospital for Children and NC Memorial Hospital. Today, the practice, Goldsboro Pediatrics, PA, provides comprehensive health services in four offices and includes fifteen pediatricians, eleven mid-level providers, a mental health professional, and two lactation consultants.

Dr. Tayloe has extensive experience in his community as a visionary leader in establishing and nourishing community-based coalitions to address school health issues, child abuse prevention, early literacy/school-readiness, Latino child health, obesity, asthma, ADHD, diabetes, and adolescent pregnancy prevention.

He helped found the Wayne Initiative for School Health (WISH) in 1997 and serves as medical director and chairperson of the board for this non-profit that operates seven school-based health centers. The WISH Centers utilize the EMR of the practice, and the practice is the overarching medical home for the 3,000 students enrolled in WISH.

Dr. Tayloe has served in the leadership of the NC Chapter of the American Academy of Pediatrics since 1983. When he was president (1993-95), North Carolina won the Outstanding Chapter Award of the AAP.

He also has held a leadership role with the national AAP since 1989 and has served on the following: Committee on State Government Affairs (1989-96); Chapter Forum Committee (1997-99; chairperson, 1999); Committee on Community Health Services (1999-2000); District IV vice-chairperson (2000-01); District chairperson (2001-07); Task Force on Immunizations (board liaison); executive committee (2007-10) and president of the AAP (2008-09); and AAP Subcommittee on Access (2011-13).

From 2010-20, Dr. Tayloe served as an AAP delegate to the American Medical Association (AMA). He was appointed to the AMA Council on Legislation (2012-20) and served as chairperson from 2019-20. He also was a member of the Governing Council of the AMA Specialty and Service Society (2017-20).

Dr. Tayloe is one of the architects of the highly successful child health system in North Carolina that included the NC Universal Childhood Vaccine Distribution Program, the physician-directed Medicaid managed care initiative, and the NC Health Choice Program (Child Health Insurance Program, or CHIP).

As a member of the American Board of Pediatrics (ABP) Strategic Planning Committee from 2003-15, he led the effort to incorporate mental health, media, and advocacy competencies into the agenda of the ABP.

Dr. Tayloe has been married to his wife, Denise, for more than fifty-one years. They have four children, all of whom are health professionals. They also have eleven wonderful grandchildren. For pleasure, Dave relaxes with family at their Pamlico River house or plays golf in Goldsboro.

## Special Acknowledgment

The Steering Committee gratefully recognizes the contributions of Micki Cabiness, Grateful Steps executive director, publisher, and friend, who guided us through the creation of Advocacy.

# Advocacy

# Part I

## The Foundation of NCPeds' Decades of Advocacy

I had no idea that advocacy would be such a critical and gratifying part of my physician role. I have learned so much from NCPeds leaders— true masters in the art of caring and the science of conviction.

# It Begins with an Email
# . . . Then the Magic Happens

**by Yun Boylston MD, FAAP**

The gratitude I have for the NC Pediatric Society (NCPeds) in truly effecting change for the children of North Carolina while giving voice to the members of our profession, runs deep. When I moved to NC after completing my residency in Texas, I had no idea that advocacy would be such a critical and gratifying part of my physician role. I have learned so much from NCPeds leaders—true masters in the art of caring and the science of conviction. Salient advocacy moments can be charted by several email threads I have been on over the years.

**EMAIL SUBJECT LINE:** BEEP BEEP PRIORITY 1

Sent by Dr. Christoph Diasio, April 2016

Impassioned, urgent—Dr. Diasio's email on behalf of President Debbie Ainsworth and the NCPeds leadership to a group of members was a five-alarm bell as we mobilized to address the Medicaid reform law passed by the NC General Assembly in 2015 that would fundamentally change the healthcare landscape and directly impact the care for half the children in our state. The email's intent was to plan a conference call (pre-Zoom) to lay out a road map for pediatric providers and garner support for the Medicaid Transformation Listening Sessions scheduled throughout the state during the upcoming weekend.

Receiving this email was pivotal for me. The society's outreach made me feel included and important, and that my actions were consequential. Up until then, I had never formally spoken in front of a broader audience regarding policy issues. I remember driving to the Guilford County Health and Human Services building after work and signing up to speak at a Listening Session. I was so nervous. How do I convey how broad political decisions will impact my patients in a way that makes people want to act? In the few minutes I had, I told personal patient stories of how undermining access to care for our patients would negatively impact the children in my community in Alamance County. I realized that out of the packed auditorium and the hundred speakers, only a handful were physicians. I then understood the power of the physician voice when we choose to use it and of the trust we are afforded by our communities.

**EMAIL SUBJECT LINE:** FRIENDS, IT IS TIME TO GET
PAID FOR AFFORDABLE CARE ACT (ACA) 90472,4!

**Sent by Dr. Graham Barden, November 2016**

Dr. Barden's email to a group of independent pediatric providers was the beginning of a two-year "David versus Goliath" legal battle for the ages that resulted in an epic win for all pediatric and family medicine providers who administer vaccines in our state. This initial email was provided as a brief update on the progress he, Dr. Christoph Diasio, and Dr. Joey Ponzi, a pediatric champion and attorney with Brooks Pierce, had made in the arduous process of resolving a statutory payment error by NC Department of Health and Human Services (DHHS) administrators regarding underpayment of vaccine administration codes during a two-year timeframe dictated by the ACA. With the support of NCPeds and the NC Academy of Family Physicians, this email, as far as Burlington Pediatrics and I were concerned, set the course for a small group of pediatric providers with limited resources but a wealth of ingenuity, chutzpah, and policy chops to take on the state.

Even within my group, wiser colleagues tempered the mood, noting nothing like this had been undertaken before. While taking a stand on principle was important, I was advised that it would be foolish to expect any financial reward from this lawsuit.

I feel fortunate to have had a ringside seat in this experience. This was a "long game" where patience and methodical actions were required. I also understood the importance of collaboration and support in raising morale among colleagues. I recognized the immeasurable talents, vast network, and intimidating knowledge base of our colleagues and the pervasive collective attitude that together we can accomplish the improbable.

**EMAIL SUBJECT LINE:** REQUEST FOR SMALL BUSINESS SIGN ON–COVERAGE GAP

**Sent by Elizabeth Hudgins, NCPeds Executive Director, April 2019**

Elizabeth's emails are some of the few that do not get overlooked in my inbox, and this was no exception. The NC General Assembly had a shot at passing legislation for Medicaid expansion during the session. In concert with two strong advocacy partners, NC Child and Care4Carolina, NCPeds reached out to see if Burlington Pediatrics, as a local business in Alamance County, would sign on to support this initiative. What started as a small business taking a stand led to connecting with the Alamance Chamber of Commerce to amplify the call for Medicaid expansion from the business community. With NC Child's policy support and insightful local data on the potential impact of closing the Medicaid gap in Alamance County, the chamber's board chair, Lisa Pennington, chamber President Mac Williams, and I sponsored a chamber resolution in support of Medicaid expansion, which passed with resounding support. As a result of this collaborative work with NC Child, Lisa was invited to participate on behalf of the chamber at Governor Cooper's small-business roundtable discussion on Medicaid.

While Medicaid expansion is still elusive in NC, the connections that stemmed from this experience are strong and lasting. Recognizing and understanding the work of our community partners like NC Child, who are aligned and poised to complement our efforts, is empowering. We celebrate the wins, but Medicaid expansion and other advocacy goals yet to be realized are also humbling reminders that we still have more work to do. I am looking forward to future emails!

## Infrastructure of NCPeds

by Elizabeth Hudgins, MPP

Throughout the decades, NCPeds has developed the infrastructure necessary to support multiple successful advocacy efforts.

### LEGAL AND TAX FRAMEWORK

At the time of its formation in 1931, the NCPeds was an informal organization of pediatric colleagues who gathered for pediatric education and social functions. After 1983, when the organization contracted with its first registered lobbyist, NCPeds registered formally as a 501(c)(6)—a membership-based nonprofit organization that exists to promote its members' business interests. As such, it enjoyed a federal tax exemption and other benefits; however, contributions were not tax-deductible for an individual's tax return, only as business expenses.

Before 1998, presidents served three-year terms, and their administrative support was a part-time secretary at the NC Medical Society. Because of the dedication and determination of early leaders, and the liaison committee/lobbyist infrastructure, NCPeds made great strides with its advocacy efforts. As the advocacy agenda grew, the presidency could become a full-time job in addition to the practice commitments of the volunteer leader.

In 1998, the leadership took the leap of faith to establish a free-standing office and to hire a full-time executive director to assure the survival and growth of its advocacy program. NCPeds did not have the funding to do all this within its current expense budget, but did have enough reserve funds to make the transition possible.

The decision to hire its own full-time executive director and establish its own office meant that dues alone would not be sufficient to cover NCPeds' operating costs. The Executive Committee made the decision to form an affiliated 501(c)(3) foundation, assuming that it would enhance non-dues revenue: contributions to the foundation

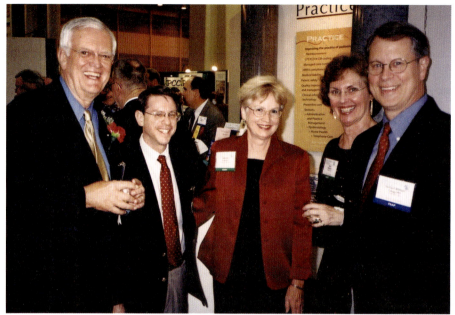

**President's reception of the AAP National Conference and Exhibition 2005, celebrating Steve Edwards as the Incoming Academy President.**

**Left to Right: Steve Edwards, Bob Schwartz, Rebecca Schwartz, Sylvia Edwards, Herb Clegg**

would be incentivized because they would be tax-deductible for individuals; and the foundation would become eligible to apply for a wide range of grants, facilitating the charitable work of the chapter and covering a portion of administrative costs. Both assumptions proved true.

As new staff members were hired to implement grants, their costs were covered by grant funds; executive director salary and other administrative costs were shared between the 501(c)(3) and the 501(c)(6). Each arm had its own board, with several overlapping positions.

During a grant-funded strategic planning project (2013-2014), the decision was made to sunset the 501(c)(6), establish NCPeds as a 501(c)(3) with an (h) election, rebrand the society as NCPeds, develop a new mission statement, and restructure the board to include directors who were not pediatricians but whose credentials and experiences made them valuable lay members.

## LEADERSHIP

Currently, the board of directors of NCPeds consists of twelve members and three lay leaders of partner organizations. Members of NCPeds elect the executive committee, which consists of the president, vice president, secretary, and treasurer, to two-year terms. Other directors also serve two-year terms and can serve a maximum of four years. Directors are elected by the board. The president and vice president also represent NCPeds within the national AAP and must be pediatricians. Other board members include practice managers and community members. The bylaws stipulate that board membership be between nine and fifteen directors.

NCPeds tries to make sure there are representatives of the private practice community, academic centers, the practice managers, and community members on the board, and that NCPeds meets standards for leadership diversity in terms of race, ethnicity, gender, geography, and other considerations.

In addition, we retain a strong working relationship with past presidents, including dinners and get-togethers to help share informal learning, leadership strategies, and fun. To help identify and recruit future leaders, we rely on meetings and committee service. Currently, approximately fifty members serve on NCPed's committees, with about forty members representing NCPeds within external commissions and groups.

At the same time the society hired its first executive director, it reduced the term of service for the president from three to two years. There were two factors that led the organization to make these changes:

1. Concern that busy pediatricians, who wanted to participate in the leadership of NCPeds, would consider the presidency an unrealistic commitment of time. The advocacy successes of NCPeds meant the organization needed dedicated leaders to assure survival of an array of excellent children's programs, while moving forward with new advocacy projects. The leaders of NCPeds have given unselfishly of their time and talents since the establishment of the organization in 1931, but these leaders must have time to make a living at their "day jobs."

2. The realization that more women were entering the profession of pediatrics and that their family and practice commitments would make it extremely difficult for them to participate in the leadership of NCPeds.

## OPEN FORUM MEETING SCHEDULE AND LOCATIONS

The leadership convenes open forum sessions in the winter, spring, and late summer; the late-summer meetings are during the annual meetings of NCPeds. Locations rotate around the state. Some meetings have been conducted virtually, especially during the COVID-19 pandemic.

**OPEN FORUM SESSIONS**

The president facilitates the presentations and discussions during in-person open forum sessions that can attract sixty to 150 pediatricians, practice managers, students, residents, government administrators, and other child advocates. Open forum agenda items may include: NCPeds operational issues, business, practice management topics, continuing medical education (CME) sessions, child advocacy topics presented by special guests, government topics presented by guest presenters from within state government, and presentations by other consultants. The spring open forum is often virtual, with the winter open forum and annual meeting occurring in-person.

**EXECUTIVE COMMITTEE AND BOARD MEETINGS**

Board meetings occur quarterly (before each open forum and during a spring retreat). The executive committee may meet prior to the board meeting. The executive committee has power to act for the board with time-sensitive issues. Most NCPeds' committees also meet quarterly and report highlights during board meetings.

**ANNUAL MEETING**

The annual meeting occurs in late summer, and the location varies from mountains to coast to the middle of the state. The meetings are typically Thursday through Sunday, with a board meeting on Thursday; a past-presidents' dinner Thursday night; an open forum Friday morning; and CME presentations Friday afternoon, Saturday, and Sunday morning. Practice managers typically meet Friday and Saturday. There is also a resident poster session, generally on Saturdays. These poster sessions involve students and residents from all five of our children's hospitals to encourage the next generation of pediatricians to attend NCPeds meetings going forward.

**OTHER EVENTS, MEETINGS, AND COMMITTEES**

In addition to the annual meeting and two additional open forums, NCPeds also typically holds a spring retreat for practice managers and White Coat Wednesday Advocacy Day, open to all members. NCPeds also traditionally has two career days—one for PL2 (second year) and one for PL3 (third year) residents. The PL3 day is in conjunction with a career fair.

In addition to the past-presidents' dinner and in conjunction with the annual meeting, past presidents are invited to the board dinner following in-person board meetings to help assure continued knowledge sharing, leadership development, and camaraderie. NCPeds benefits greatly from the continued involvement of its dedicated past presidents.

NCPeds also serves as a convener for the Child Health Insurance Coalition, consisting of mostly child health advocates. In addition, most of NCPeds' ten other committees are staffed and meet at least quarterly, typically virtually. NCPeds also has a number of special topic-oriented task forces (such as child abuse, Medicaid reform, race equity, and climate change), which are also supported by staff. The committees help grow and inform the leadership pipeline for NCPeds.

## ADVOCACY

As a 501(c)(3), NCPeds can use chapter resources to lobby and advocate for child-health issues. However, we cannot in any way support or oppose candidates for office. In 1983, the first lobbyist was signed to a retainer agreement with NCPeds. The lobbyist represents NCPeds at the NC General Assembly, provides guidance to the executive director and policy committee, and may present at NCPeds events. The current lobbyist provides both consultation and lobbying services. The executive director is also a registered lobbyist. NCPeds works to build avenues for communication with key government administrative leaders as well, including having regular meetings with the leaders and inviting the leaders to be presenters during open forum sessions. NCPeds members and staff also offer a child-health perspective to a number of statewide committees and task forces.

## STAFF

Since 1998, NCPeds has had a full-time executive director and an office in the state capital. The executive committee hires the executive director, and the executive director hires other staff, based upon available resources and current NCPeds needs. Staff help implement board direction for membership, finance, grant writing, grant implementation, events, policy, and other priorities.

Current staff consists of seven full-time employees, including operations staff of:
- a full-time executive director,
- a membership services and events manager,
- a part-time finance manager, and
- a part-time fundraising and membership specialist.

NCPeds is also home to the Fostering Health NC initiative, which seeks to link children and youth in foster care statewide with strong, trauma-informed medical homes. This state grant fully covers the cost of the program director and two implementation specialists.

## FINANCE AND DEVELOPMENT COMMITTEE

The finance and development committee is usually co-chaired by the treasurer and another leader designated by the president. The NCPeds president approves the appointment of other members of the finance and development committee to oversee and monitor finances. The treasurer and key staff set the agenda for this committee so current budget issues can be addressed in a timely fashion and so members and practices are encouraged to donate money, above and beyond membership dues, to supplement NCPeds operating funds. An NCPeds Legacy Fund with the NC Community Foundation has been initiated so members can designate NCPeds as the recipient of many types of charitable donations, including estate funds.

## COMMUNICATION

In 1990, George Engstrom, MD, FAAP, a community pediatrician in Concord and a talented and creative writer, was recruited to become the first NCPeds newsletter editor. Dr. Engstrom took this responsibility off the plate of the president and took

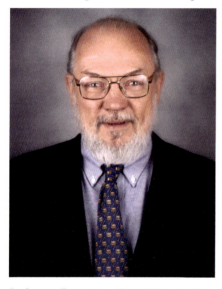

Dr. George Engstrom, editor of the popular *North Carolina Pediatrician* newsletter

the monthly "snail mail" communication to members to the next level. He recruited members to write articles concerning important topics and created an avenue for students, residents, and young pediatricians to make contributions to this much-improved newsletter. NCPeds now has a part-time consultant for media and communication who writes our newsletter and works to garner earned media coverage, as appropriate. NCPeds also has a number of social media accounts, including Facebook, Twitter, and Instagram. There is a member "push" listserv where staff and leadership share information with approximately 2,300 members at least weekly. The open rate for emails from this listserv is about twice the industry average.

There is also a highly active iterative practice manager listserv that troubleshoots problems and serves as an early warning system to identify problems of everyday practice such as Medicaid managed care payment issues and vaccines and, more recently, COVID-19.

## SOLUTION SHARE

During the COVID-19 pandemic, NCPeds began convening weekly thirty-minute virtual forums, at 5:30 p.m. every Tuesday, so leadership could offer support to members and so members could share issues with leadership that need attention from state government administrators and leaders. The leadership arranges for periodic presentations by selected government administrators/leaders and/or pediatrician

# NCPeds has relied on its strong relationships with agency officials, elected leaders, and non-profit leaders to craft, promote, and implement needed regulations and policies.

specialists so participants could learn from experts. Participants could also explain their troubles to experts during the pandemic. Usually twenty to thirty members or guests participated in these Solution Share forums. These Zoom events have continued after the public health emergency and are much appreciated by members. Topics have included Medicaid transformation, Children's Health Insurance Program (CHIP)-Medicaid merger, COVID-19 vaccine commercialization, minor's consent, opioid education requirements, infant formula shortages, oral health, and other issues of importance.

### AWARDS: CREDITING OUR CHAMPIONS

Throughout the years, NCPeds has relied on its strong relationships with agency officials, elected leaders, and non-profit leaders to craft, promote, and implement needed regulations and policies and to pass child-, family-, and pediatrician-friendly legislation. Therefore, recognizing and celebrating our successes and crediting those who made them possible have been critical components of our advocacy program.

NCPeds honors deserving advocacy partners and members with a variety of awards. These are presented at one of its regular meetings. There is usually a business luncheon during the annual meeting for the purpose of recognizing as many awardees as possible. These awards often create a lasting bond between recipients and NCPeds, and further promote working together to improve the well-being of children and their families in addition to ensuring all children have access to well-educated, caring child-health professionals.

Some awards given in honor of important people who have assisted NCPeds in its advocacy work:
- David Tayloe Sr., MD, FAAP: President, 1980-83; (see *Big Dave: Visionary Leader*)
- Floyd Denny, MD, FAAP: Chief of Pediatrics at UNC (1960-1981)
- Samuel Katz, MD, FAAP: Chief of Pediatrics at Duke (1968-1990)
- Jimmy Simon, MD, FAAP: Chief of Pediatrics at Wake Forest (1974-1996)

- Jon Tingelstad, MD, FAAP: Chief of Pediatrics at East Carolina (1977-2000)
- James Bernstein: Founder of the Office of Rural Health Resources in the NC Department of Health and Human Services and creator of the Community Care of NC Medicaid program (1973-2005)
- Steve Shore, MSW: Executive Director of NCPeds (1999-2014)
- Tom Vitaglione, MPH: A respected and trusted friend of children in multiple roles in the NC Department of Health and Human Services, including head of Children's Services in the Division of Public Health (1970-2000); senior fellow for NC Child (2000-present)

NCPeds Award recipients from 1987-2022 are found in the NCPeds Awards section following the Appendix.

## Liaison Committee to Open Forum

by Jane Meschan Foy, MD, FAAP; Steve Shore, MSW

The authors of this publication inherited organizational infrastructure from presidents who led NCPeds during the 1960s, especially Will London, MD, FAAP, and John (Jack) Lynch, MD, FAAP. From the beginning, NCPeds has been blessed with incredible volunteer leadership of general and academic pediatricians, some serving in leadership roles for more than twenty years!

The liaison committee emerged as a powerful engagement concept. Originally, the president invited pediatricians from across the state to attend liaison committee meetings in three locations at the time of the tri-annual executive committee meetings—winter, spring, and late summer. As of 2014, the NCPeds Executive Committee was reorganized to a board structure. The late-summer liaison committee meeting occurred during the NCPeds Annual Meeting. As new presidents assumed their roles, they could add more pediatricians to the invitation list.

All liaison committee members received "snail mail" notice of the meetings, and attendance varied but averaged about fifty members. With the advent of Medicaid, it became clear that pediatricians needed to work with state government leaders to develop a Medicaid program that could work for children, families, and primary care professionals. Therefore, key state government administrators and leaders began to receive invitations to make presentations and to engage attendees in discussions during liaison committee meetings. Over time, non-physician child advocates were also invited to attend. These meetings occurred on the mornings following evening executive committee meetings, usually on Fridays or Saturdays such that liaison committee meetings occurred on Saturday or Sunday. NCPeds paid for breakfast and lunch to encourage attendance. For the late-summer annual meeting, the executive

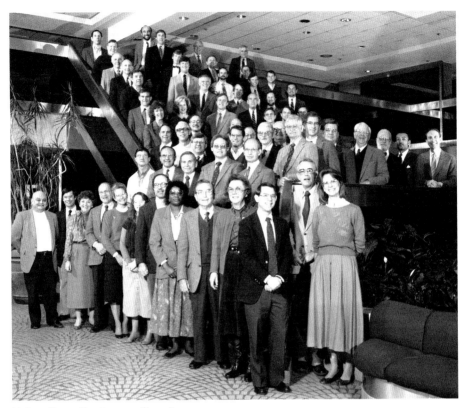

**Liaison Committee became Open Forum**

committee convened on Thursday, with the liaison committee meeting on Friday morning, immediately before the beginning of the annual pediatric education sessions. NCPeds committees often scheduled meetings to coincide with the approximate time and location of liaison committee meetings.

Wally Brown, MD, FAAP, general pediatrician in Raleigh and member of both the executive and liaison committees during a long stretch of his career, reflected on the value of the liaison committee:

> Look at the outcomes of some of our NCPeds campaigns—those outcomes were possible because of the networking and teamwork that emanate from liaison committee meetings. If you write down the outcomes for three of those major campaigns—immunizations, Medicaid, CHIP (named NC Health Choice)—you can trace the basis for those outcomes back to the infrastructure/networking of the liaison committee.

**Immunizations:** All children receive all recommended vaccines in all primary health care settings with no financial barriers for families of all children; child-health professionals receive fair payment for giving vaccines to all children; and child-health professionals who participate in the immunization program receive liability protection.

**Medicaid:** All Medicaid-eligible children have access to comprehensive health services, including early periodic screening, diagnosis, and treatment (EPSDT), in all primary care health care settings. Child-health professionals receive fair payment for services rendered to Medicaid-eligible patients. These patients have access to all necessary treatment services/materials/equipment, according to clinical guidelines agreed upon by leaders of child-health professional organizations and Medicaid.

**CHIP, named NC Health Choice:** All CHIP-eligible children have access to comprehensive health services, including well-child care consistent with Medicaid's EPSDT, in all primary care settings. Child-health professionals receive fair payment for services rendered to CHIP-eligible patients. These patients have access to all necessary treatment services/materials/equipment, according to clinical guidelines agreed upon by leaders of child health professional organizations and Medicaid.

Jane Meschan Foy, MD, FAAP, started as a general pediatrician in Greensboro and Winston-Salem and then moved to the Wake Forest University Department of Pediatrics. She was president of NCPeds in 1998-99 when it made the leap of faith to establish a freestanding office and hire a full-time executive director. She commented:

We changed the name of the 'liaison committee' to the 'open forum' during my presidency mainly because some of our members, including me, thought they needed an invitation to attend. We hoped the name change, outreach to members, and addition of CME credit for some sessions would build pediatrician attendance and, in turn, enhance participation of new partners by virtue of exposing them to a larger audience of pediatricians. Our newly hired Executive Director Steve Shore noted the increased attendance, especially when CME credits became available. I recall one particularly large open forum when NC's Medicaid Director Dick Peruzzi spoke about securing support from pediatricians for the dental varnish initiative (see *Into the Mouths of Babes: A Collaborative Solution for Improving Children's Oral Health*), and, in return, we pressed for his support of our mental health initiative. Soon after, our mental health task force started holding its meetings at the Medicaid offices at the invitation of Mr. Peruzzi.

What was the value of the liaison committee meetings to the child-health system in our state? More than fifty percent of children in many areas of North Carolina live in families that cannot afford to pay for recommended comprehensive health services. Before Medicaid, these children usually received very fragmented care, bouncing from health department to hospital emergency department to primary care practices based upon the economic status of families. There was a glaring need for government leaders to develop programs that made it possible for low-income, at-risk children to receive necessary health services. The federal government created and funded immunization, Medicaid, and CHIP programs with appropriations and gave wide latitude to the states to develop programs that work for the families of eligible children and for child-health professionals.

In North Carolina, since the liaison committee was initiated, government administrators have been invited to participate in leadership meetings of NCPeds. During these meetings, government administrators learn about what child-health professionals can do to help them implement children's programs and are assured that child health professionals will participate in the programs so all eligible children receive all recommended services. Attendees are encouraged to let the government administrators know what the state government needs to do to assure universal participation of child-health professionals in government-funded/administered programs. It is understood, during these leadership meetings, that payment of child-health professionals needs to be at a level that encourages the child-health professionals to participate in the programs. At times between liaison committee/open forum meetings, NCPeds leaders often have follow-up meetings with government administrators to further develop immunization, Medicaid, and CHIP programs that work for children, families, and child-health professionals. If it is necessary to involve legislators or other government officials in the effort to create and nurture good child-health programs, child-health professionals can become involved with elected government officials in ways not possible for government administrators who attend NCPeds meetings, as administrators are state employees and cannot lobby elected officials. Since the executive committee elected to fund a full-time executive director, the open forum has included Category I CME sessions, usually scheduled after the government affairs presentations/discussions. Our academic medical centers have directed the CME program and provided speakers. NCPeds partners with the American Academy of Pediatrics (AAP) Department of Education to assure attendees can record this CME credit into their AAP transcripts. By providing CME, NCPeds is doing all that it can to assure optimal attendance at open forum meetings.

The leadership of NCPeds has always been voluntary, beginning with the individual initiative of Wilburt C. Davison, MD, chief of pediatrics and dean of the medical school at Duke University, in 1931. NCPeds does elect officers, but it is rare that it conducts a really contested election. None of the leaders receive any salary or benefits, other than travel expenses when representing the society at AAP meetings or during necessary in-state travel to represent NCPeds in key meetings/forums. NCPeds pays hotel expenses for all executive committee members, including the president and vice president, during the annual meeting of NCPeds. The executive committee hires the executive director, and the executive director hires other staff as needed and feasible.

# Early Legislative Efforts

**by Steve Edwards MD, FAAP**

NCPeds was formed in 1931 within one year of the founding of the American Academy of Pediatrics. The organization focused initially on pediatric education and social functions associated with each meeting. In 1968, President William London, MD, FAAP, led NCPeds to take a big step forward in child advocacy when he formed the liaison committee (now called open forum), an informal gathering of pediatricians representing various geographic areas of the state, department chairs of the five pediatric teaching programs in NC, and heads of state government agencies that operated child-health programs. Meetings were held in various locations in the state three to four times a year and around forty to sixty individuals attended. This forum facilitated dialogue between the three entities and nurtured a unique atmosphere for creative advances.

In 1975, Archie Johnson Jr., MD, FAAP, began his term as president for the years 1975-1978. He had recently been the first neonatologist at Wake Memorial Hospital (now named WakeMed) and had recently left that position to work in state government. He was considered an up-and-coming politico with ties to both political parties. On his office wall were signed photographs from Governor James Hunt (D) and Senator Jesse Helms (R). Dr. Johnson spearheaded the first legislative initiative of NCPeds when he led a successful effort to pass legislation to require insurance companies to provide health insurance for children from birth. Prior to this, health insurance for children began at age one month. As a neonatologist, Dr. Johnson recognized the devastating economic impact on families that had premature babies. Though Dr. Johnson carried the heavy water on this issue, he recruited members of both the NCPeds executive and liaison committees to contact legislators to promote the bill.

Concurrently in 1975, the US Congress passed Public Law (PL) 93-641, a federal law that created health planning agencies—officially called Health Systems Agencies or HSAs—in every state. Governor Holshouser and his administration decided to create six HSAs across North Carolina.

At the state level, the implementation of PL 93-641 also created a State Health Coordinating Council (SHCC) with other appointed representatives from the six regions. Governor Holshouser appointed Dr. Johnson, president of NCPeds, as the chair of the State Health Coordinating Council. David Flaherty was the secretary of the Department of Human Resources (DHR) (now the Department of Health and Human Services). The SHCC existed within the Division of Facility Services, the agency responsible for the State Medical Facilities Plan that dictated the approval of Certificates of Need (CONs) for hospital beds, nursing home beds, big equipment like the first computerized tomography (CT) scanners at the time, lithotripters, and free-standing outpatient surgical centers. Dr. Johnson was a formidable leader for the state health structure until his death in 1978.

Dave Williams, MD, FAAP, became president of NCPeds for 1978-1981. Through contacts via the liaison committee, he initiated a partnership with the NC Department of Human Resources to jointly collaborate in developing a child health plan for North Carolina (see *Membership: Key to Effective Advocacy*). Multiple pediatricians participated in meetings over a yearlong effort to develop the plan. When the plan was published in 1979, two phrases created immediate controversy: (1) "Every child should be wanted" was interpreted as "abortion approval," and (2) "Medical home" was totally misunderstood as support for taking children away from their parents. Despite exhaustive efforts to explain the language in the proposal, it was never accepted. During a heated gubernatorial race in 1980 between incumbent Democrat James Hunt and conservative Republican I. Beverly Lake, the child health plan became a political hot potato and disappeared, never to resurface.

In spite of that, many of the specific priorities in the plan were diligently achieved because they provided practical guidance for pediatricians who stepped into the spotlight of child advocacy across North Carolina.

In 1978 NCPeds, through the American Academy of Pediatrics, applied for a federal grant to compare the cost of healthcare in private offices, university clinics, and health departments. The objective was to demonstrate the cost effectiveness of the medical home. The grant was funded for five years. Jonathan Kotch, MD, FAAP, of the University of North Carolina School of Public Health was the lead investigator. Unfortunately, after one planning year, Governor Hunt sensed political vulnerability in his race for reelection and returned the grant money to Washington without ever informing NCPeds.

This series of events demonstrates there were significant obstacles as NCPeds promoted action, yet struggled to gain recognition and traction as advocates for children. Perhaps these nullified initiatives paved the way for our most significant accomplishment to date—the childhood vaccine compensation legislation (see *Big Dave: Visionary Leader*).

# The Growth of Collaboration

by Tom Vitaglione, MPH

In the mid-1970s, I became administrative head of the child health branch in the Division of Public Health. As such, I was invited to one of the initial meetings of the NCPeds' liaison committee. This was a new approach to bringing together practicing pediatricians, academic pediatric leaders, and members of state government to explore issues of mutual interest.

I expected a professional organization meeting devoted almost exclusively to advancing the financial status of pediatric practitioners. I was wrong. Most of the meeting focused on improving the health and well-being of children, not only through the enhanced practice of care, but also prevention through family and community

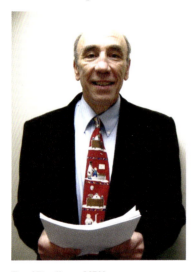

**Tom Vitaglione, MPH**

education. I immediately felt at home and sensed the potential of this new relationship to make a real difference in the lives of children and families. I was right.

Almost invariably, pediatricians are trusted and respected members of their communities. Their voices carry gravitas, especially when it becomes clear that they are advocating not for their own financial well-being, but for child and family well-being. Thus, any campaign to improve child health and safety is immensely helped by the involvement of the pediatric community.

Most of the articles in this book reflect the successes achieved by bringing together state government, NCPeds, and community advocates (including community pediatricians). Through the past forty years, this coalition has played a critical role in improving child health and safety on countless fronts. These include the expansion of newborn screening and childhood immunization, virtually all child passenger safety statutes, the implementation of expanded health insurance coverage through NC Health Choice (SCHIP), the elimination of corporal punishment in the public schools, and the list could go on and on.

The reputation of NCPeds has grown to the point that its endorsement of any child health/safety proposal is critical. Legislators respond more quickly and positively to pediatricians in their constituencies. The beneficiaries are children and families.

This systematic collaboration between state government, NCPeds, and the overall advocacy community has become institutionalized in our state. One hopes that this model will be adopted elsewhere across the nation.

# Big Dave: Visionary Leader
**by Dave Tayloe Jr., MD, FAAP**

I began my solo practice in Goldsboro, in July 1977, and my pediatrician father, known to most as "Big Dave," immediately invited me (known to all my family as "Little Dave") to the annual meeting of NCPeds and my first experience as the

newest member of the liaison committee. My dad had been a member of NCPeds since his days in pediatric residency at Duke University and could remember early meetings in a hotel in Roaring Gap that ended up with an all-night adult beverage experience in the hotel room of Wilburt C. Davison, MD, FAAP, chief of pediatrics and dean of the medical school at Duke.

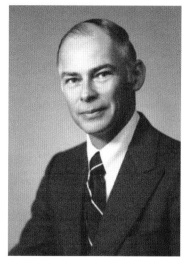

David T. Tayloe Sr., MD, FAAP

Big Dave was so important because our rich advocacy foundation became a big-time reality for all of us when he was found liable in a diphtheria-tetanus-pertussis (DTaP) vaccine-related injury lawsuit in 1985. He was probably the most respected pediatrician in the state at that time. He was born David Thomas Tayloe, destined to become the fourth generation of physicians since Civil War days in Washington, North Carolina, population 10,000. His parents died when he was a young teenager, so he was raised by very devoted aunts and uncles. He entered UNC undergraduate school in 1942, in the middle of World War II, and did so well on a screening test that he was not drafted into military service but allowed to complete his college courses and get his MD at the University of Pennsylvania School of Medicine. By the time he finished medical school, I was two years old, and he had to serve his "military time" while doing a rotating internship at the Medical College of Virginia and his pediatric residency at Duke. In 1955, he returned to Washington, where he established Washington Pediatrics in a three-bedroom house on a dirt street just one block north of the Tayloe Hospital and School of Nursing. He was probably the first board-certified pediatrician to set up practice east of Raleigh and was committed to the "medical home" concept long before the AAP adopted it as the gold standard for community practice. He took care of every child who came through the door of his office, and worked closely with the health department, the department of social services, and the public schools to assure his patients received the services they needed, before there was a Medicaid (1965) or State Child Health Insurance Program (SCHIP, 1998). And there were no health insurance plans that paid for outpatient pediatric care at the time.

Dr. Davison made sure my dad became involved in the NC Pediatric Society while he was completing his pediatric residency at Duke. Big Dave served as president of NCPeds in 1972 and again from 1981 to 1983. In 1981, he led the effort to win the AAP Outstanding Large Chapter (chapters with over 300 members) Award. He wrote this commentary for the chapter newsletter explaining the AAP honor:

> In October of 1981, the North Carolina Chapter of the American Academy of Pediatrics was judged the best large chapter in North America. This rewarded a successful effort on the part of the chapter for excellence. Many members and leaders over the years unselfishly contributed.
>
> This organization was started by an academician to gather together physicians primarily involved in the care of children. In the beginning, our efforts were educational and social. As time went on, we became a chapter of the American Academy of Pediatrics. Three new four-year medical schools became a part of the scene. Each of them enthusiastically contributed to the strength of the group. Government agencies, both federal and state, became increasingly more involved in children's programs. Child care physicians from these government agencies eagerly supported the organization. More than any other factor, the willing cooperation and communication among practitioners, academicians, and government-based physicians insured success.
>
> At the present time, practitioners from approved residency training programs significantly enhance child care in this state. Sophisticated tertiary care in the medical centers backs up the primary care of pediatricians and provides dynamic leadership. The various government agencies are charged with the overall public health responsibilities of pediatrics. In addition, through their several agencies, they administer financial help to disadvantaged children.
>
> Accomplishment, building, learning, and providing are all of extreme importance, but "lest the world be too much with us," we must always cultivate that innocent, joyful, enthusiasm of youth that is so compellingly attractive to all of us.

*– David T. Tayloe Sr., MD*
*Washington, NC; 05-21-1982*

During his term as president, he convinced the executive committee to contract with a legislative lobbying firm and a public relations company so NCPeds would have the services of those important allies going forward. He developed an excellent working relationship with the director of Medicaid and the secretary of Human Resources (later Health and Human Services). He and the past president of the NCPeds, Dave Williams, MD, FAAP, met with the governor on a regular basis. In 1983, while he was president, NCPeds developed a key contact legislative telephone tree so that every one of our 120 legislators was assigned to a pediatrician for legislative lobbying purposes. Thus, NCPeds had many vital components for a successful legislative lobbying initiative by 1983—all we needed was a crisis so that we could prove our value to the state's children, families, and physicians!

He was committed to the "medical home" concept long before the AAP adopted it as the gold standard.

In 1982, a news special from Great Britain, depicting eleven young children who had supposedly suffered brain damage from the pertussis vaccine, appeared on national television in our country. Based upon this dramatic news story, attorneys immediately began to advertise their services concerning potential lawsuits against physicians and vaccine manufacturers. It would not be until 2006 that scientists would discover a genetic cause (Dravet Syndrome) for nine of the eleven children. No link between pertussis vaccine and permanent brain damage has ever been scientifically proven.

In 1985, Big Dave was found legally at fault for medical malpractice during a jury trial in Wilmington, North Carolina, in a case involving a child who received the pertussis vaccine from his pediatrician partner's nurse in 1974. This child was brought into the courtroom to show the jury that he suffered with developmental disability and seizures. The jury awarded the family $3.5 million; my father and his partner had $1.4 million in medical malpractice insurance in 1974.

NCPeds convened a regularly scheduled liaison committee meeting in Pinehurst, North Carolina, three days after my father's verdict became public knowledge. Secretary of Health and Human Services Phil Kirk, a Republican, attended that momentous open forum in Pinehurst. A large group of pediatricians attended to express their outrage about my father's situation. NCPeds committed to work with Secretary Kirk to address the problem. Pediatricians made it clear to the secretary that pediatricians could not continue giving vaccines to children in this litigious environment. Our practice stopped giving the pertussis component of the DTP vaccine, giving all our patients DT (diphtheria-tetanus) instead.

As a member of the executive committee, I was appointed chair of an ad-hoc committee on vaccine liability. I was passionate about doing something to both vindicate my father and to assure that pediatricians could continue to participate in the immunization program. I was introduced to the new young lobbyist of NCPeds, Henry Jones, from Raleigh. Henry and I met with the secretary and my local member of the state house of representatives, a pharmacist, in the secretary's office in Raleigh on the Monday after the liaison committee meeting. Secretary Kirk had worked for a member of the US House of Representatives in the recent past and that congressman had helped develop a federal vaccine injury compensation program bill supported by the larger AAP. The secretary provided guidance to us as we developed state legislation to compensate children who had possibly been permanently injured by state-mandated vaccines, to protect physicians and manufacturers from vaccine-related injury lawsuits, to prevent severe escalation of vaccine costs from the medico-legal crisis, and to assure a pathway for punishment of providers or manufacturers proven to have wantonly and willfully caused permanent injury to a patient during their participation in the vaccine program. We recruited trial lawyers in the House and Senate to lead our legislative campaign. We met repeatedly with representatives of Lederle Labs, the major manufacturer of the DTP vaccine, and the "deepest pocket" for any vaccine-related injury lawsuit.

In July 1986, the legislature passed the NC Childhood Vaccine Injury Compensation Program law that accomplished all our objectives. Families of children thought to have been injured by state-mandated vaccines could apply to the Industrial Commission of NC, much like workers' compensation applicants, and the industrial commission would utilize a table of compensable events prepared by infectious disease experts in the academic medical centers of the state to decide if a given child could possibly have suffered a compensable event from a vaccine. If so, the commission would grant the child an award based upon predicted life-long expenses calculated by professional actuaries. Physicians and vaccine manufacturers were shielded from jury trials but could be investigated by the NC Attorney General to determine if a party had committed wanton and willful negligence in each case. The state could remove the medical license of a negligent provider or levy a fine on an unethical manufacturer.

NC became the first state to ever pass legislation to establish such a program. The federal government passed similar legislation, creating the National Vaccine Program, in late 1986. There really was no evidence that the NC experience influenced the federal legislative process, although AAP representatives did visit the state during our 1985–86 legislative campaign. I was clueless at the time as to what the AAP was doing to address vaccine liability.

During the legislative campaign, a pharmaceutical company donated $5,000 to NCPeds to help defray lobbying costs. After the campaign, NCPeds sent out requests for voluntary donations of twenty-five dollars from members, and eighty-five percent of the membership sent in money. NCPeds won the Outstanding Large Chapter award from the AAP mostly because of this successful advocacy project.

During this vaccine liability crisis, vaccine prices skyrocketed. I paid fifteen cents for a dose of DTP vaccine in 1980. By 1990, I was paying at least ten dollars per dose. Physicians were not being paid by health insurance plans or Medicaid to give vaccines; vaccine costs were bundled into fees for well-child visits. Many families were unable to afford to have their children immunized in physicians' offices and did not always take their children to the health department for free state-funded vaccines. Therefore, in 1986 NCPeds developed an appropriations bill calling for the legislature to fund vaccines for all the children in our state, making sure physicians could continue giving vaccines in their practices. The price tag for this bill was about $2.5 million per year.

The chapter worked on this until Governor Jim Hunt, at the insistence of future Secretary of Health and Human Services David Bruton, MD, a pediatrician, convinced the legislature to appropriate $16 million per year (the price tag went up significantly between 1986 and 1994 because new vaccines were added to the list of state-mandated vaccines for children) to establish the NC Childhood Universal Vaccine Distribution Program in 1994. Through this program, all physicians in NC who participated in the program could receive vaccines for all their patients free-of-charge from the immunization branch.

In 1993, the federal government created the Vaccines for Children (VFC) program, whereby the federal government would pay for all vaccines needed by children on Medicaid, uninsured children, Native American children, and Alaskan Eskimo children. Federal VFC funding allowed our legislature to reduce the state appropriation for the universal program by fifty percent. The federal government, within VFC, permitted state Medicaid programs to establish vaccine administration fees so that physicians could be paid for their vaccine services. NCPeds worked with the Commission on Health Services of NC to assure our physicians received the maximum allowable fee for vaccine administration ($13.71 per vaccine).

With the combined effects of the state's universal program and Vaccines for Children, immunization rates in our state rose to all-time highs despite lingering vaccine liability concerns, an increase in the number of vaccines recommended for children, and rising vaccine prices. Therefore, the NCPeds had turned a disastrous situation in 1985 into amazing progressive changes for our state so that children, families, and physicians could assure optimal immunization of our children.

This was largely possible because Big Dave was such an important personality in pediatrics in the state and because he had helped establish the NCPeds infrastructure that supported the major legislative lobbying effort needed to address the vaccine liability crisis.

I needed Big Dave's lobbyist to figure out how to develop and pass tort reform legislation. I was a 36-year-old rural pediatrician with no government affairs experience. My passion for the cause, my energy, and the innate intelligence necessary to be accepted into medical school would not have allowed me to accomplish my legislative goals without the assistance of a skillful, dedicated lobbyist. We used Big Dave's public relations firm to get our story into the news when anti-vaccine rhetoric was winning the day. We needed key contact pediatricians to make sure legislators understood the relationship of our tort reform legislation to the overall health of our state. We needed pediatricians who had attended liaison committee meetings and understood the importance of physicians working with government entities to promote excellent health programs for children in all our communities. Big Dave helped give us all these key tools so that we could actually develop and pass meaningful legislation during a major crisis for the state's children, families, and physicians.

During this time frame, NCPeds established the Dave Tayloe Sr. Award, which is given annually to honor a pediatrician who has gone above and beyond to emulate the outgoing approach to pediatrics of Big Dave. In 1991, it was my privilege to present the first Dave Tayloe Sr. Award to a young pediatrician in Asheville, Andrea Gravatt, for her tireless work in the field of child abuse.

## Medicaid Reform: Negotiating with State Government

by Steve Edwards, MD, FAAP

I joined the AAP Council on Pediatric Practice (COPP) in 1977. In reviewing the materials for a COPP meeting, I was surprised by data revealing the high cost-per-patient encounters of health departments around our country. I began to consider an alternative. Why not transfer much of this care to private pediatricians who could offer excellent cost-effective care to all but the most developmentally and medically complex children?

The biggest impediment was the well-established fact that financial compensation through Medicaid was too low to have fiscally viable practices for pediatricians who saw high percentages of Medicaid patients. The obvious answer would be to raise Medicaid payment rates, but efforts to accomplish this had been fruitless.

One night after a COPP dinner, I discussed this concern with Tom Robb, an AAP staffer for COPP. Tom offered to help write a proposal to Health and Human

Services (HHS) for a study to compare the cost and quality of delivering Medicaid services in private practices with services in both health departments and pediatric academic centers. Tom did most of the heavy lifting as they prepared and submitted the proposal.

Amazingly, it was accepted and funded for five years! Dr. Jonathan Kotch of the UNC Pediatric Department would be the lead investigator. The first year would be consumed by setting up the program, and then data would be collected for four years. Unfortunately, after the first year, North Carolina Governor James Hunt got involved in a heated re-election campaign in which health care financing was an issue, and returned the remainder of the grant money to HHS without any discussions with pediatricians.

Soon after assuming his role as president of NCPeds in 1981, Dr. David T. Tayloe, Sr. held a planning session one cold winter weekend in Greensboro. Ten to twelve pediatricians attended. It is from this meeting that the idea for hiring Henry Jones, a lobbyist, and Epley Associates, a public relations firm, emerged. Less remembered is the decision to merge all

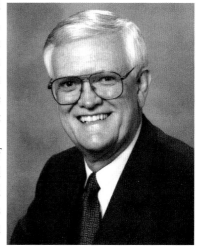

Steve Edwards, MD, FAAP

committees associated with the government into a single organization called the Government Programs Committee. I was to chair the coordinated group, and each committee continued to function as usual with the expectation that we were to coordinate activities. NCPeds committees included: Crippled Children's Program (Title V), Medicaid, WIC (Women and Infant Care), and others.

I also served as chair of the NCPeds Medicaid Committee. In that capacity I met regularly with Barbara Matula, who headed that section in the NC Department of Human Resources. She had several pediatric associates including Drs. Jimmie Rhyne and Lewis Bock—both excellent pediatricians and fine people. I believed strongly that improving Medicaid reimbursement was the key to improved access to health care for poor children. I became frustrated with the lack of progress.

Other pediatricians and I continued to meet three or four times a year with Medicaid administrators. Occasionally we were able to gain small fee raises, but none were of the magnitude that would make Medicaid viable for practices to care for a high percentage of Medicaid patients. Dr. David Tayloe, Sr. referred to pediatricians who saw large numbers of Medicaid patients as "medical missionaries." Medicaid administrator comments during most meetings went something like this: "Pediatricians are such nice people. We appreciate your work and would like to increase reimbursement, but there just isn't any money." In time, I could see that hospitals, pharmacies, and other provider groups were managing to get increases, but pediatricians were only receiving periodic token fee upgrades that did not cover inflationary costs of practices. At the liaison committee, I floated the possibility of a Medicaid boycott and received zero support from the pediatric community.

In the meantime, I completed my term on COPP, and in 1984 was appointed to the AAP Council on Government Affairs (COGA). Dr. Dave Tayloe, Jr. joined a new AAP Provisional Committee on State Legislation (PCOSL) and became the chairperson of PCOSL for NCPeds in 1985 during the vaccine liability crisis.

Dave and I were in positions to appreciate the "Equal Access" provision in the Omnibus Budget Reconciliation Act of 1989 (OBRA-89) that stated that "Payments for Medicaid services should be such that Medicaid patients should have the same access to care as other patients in the same geographic area." The Pennsylvania Chapter hopped on this immediately and began a legal challenge to their state.

> I believed strongly that improving Medicaid reimbursement was the key to improved access to health care for poor children. I became frustrated with the lack of progress.

By 1990, I was the incoming NCPeds president; Dr. Dave Tayloe, Jr. was vice-president; and Dr. Wallace "Wally" Brown served as chairperson of the NCPeds Medicaid Committee. When Barbara Matula became director of Medicaid in 1979, Drs. Dave Williams, Dave Tayloe, Sr., and others met with her and her staff of pediatricians regularly to address ways to make Medicaid more user-friendly for pediatricians and to ask for fair payment for pediatricians who participate in Medicaid. When the OBRA-89 was signed into law at the federal level, it called for fair payment in Medicaid to assure that Medicaid patients had equal access to physicians. Ms. Matula correctly quipped, "There's not a single state in compliance with this!" From the creation of Medicaid, states had been allowed to set payment at any percentage of Medicare that fit their budgets; no state was paying physicians 100 percent of the Medicare rates.

NCPeds leaders took the OBRA-89 issue to the NCPeds Executive Committee. There was strong support for pressing ahead with the development of a document that could become the basis for bringing legal action against the state for not paying physicians who participate in Medicaid fairly, based upon the language of OBRA-89. Henceforth, attorney Henry Jones, NCPeds lobbyist, and his associate, Steve Shaber, joined us at each Medicaid meeting. These attorneys began to draft documents that could be utilized by the chapter to bring an Equal Access lawsuit against the state. From that point on, every meeting with Ms. Matula and/or her staff was attended by Wally, Dave, and me, plus two or three other pediatricians and our lawyers. Ms. Matula always had implied that her team wanted Medicaid raises but that superiors prevented it. At one meeting early in negotiations, I asked her, "Would it be helpful if we sued you?" After a hesitant pause, Ms. Matula practically shouted "NO."

Our goal had been Medicaid payments equal to those in Medicare. After two or three more meetings over a period of around six months, Ms. Matula offered to increase payments by 30 percent. This was about 15 percent short of Medicare parity. When we took this to our executive committee, there was staunch support for acceptance and putting plans for a lawsuit on hold. The executive committee chose a wait-and-see course based upon the significant increase in payment offered by Ms. Matula.

In 1994, Dr. Brown negotiated doubling the compensation to pediatricians for Early and Periodic Screening, Diagnosis, and Treatment (EPSDT) visits, the well-child encounters recommended from birth to age twenty-one years for Medicaid-eligible children. When the Vaccines for Children Program was implemented in 1994, Dr. Dave Tayloe, Jr. and Dr. Harry Smith negotiated the maximum federally-allowed payment for vaccine administration fees for North Carolina physicians. In the late 1990s, when pediatrician David Bruton, MD, headed the NC Department of Human Resources, payments for Medicaid visits were raised to parity with Medicare.

In the late 1990s, the Oklahoma AAP Chapter sued its state under OBRA-89. After the chapter spent several hundred thousand dollars on litigation, their district court threw out the case, ruling that the chapter lacked standing to bring the case.

Our methodical negotiating slowly yielded results, thanks to the infrastructure of NCPeds and the wisdom of its leaders!

## Membership: Key to Effective Advocacy

by Dave Williams, MD, FAAP; Steve Shore, MSW

I served as president of the NC Pediatric Society from 1978–1980. I believe that three factors were instrumental in setting a new direction for NCPeds: the work done by leadership in the late 1970s and early 1980s to revive the liaison committee hosted by the officers with our standing committee chairs and attended by many individual

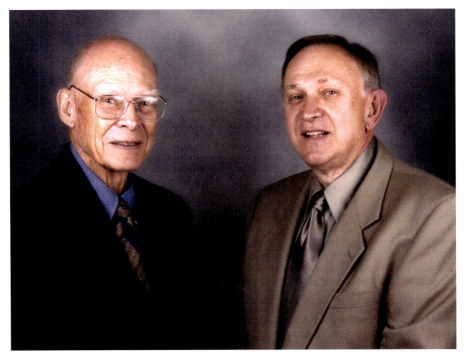

**Dave Tayloe Sr., MD, FAAP, and Dave Williams MD, FAAP**

members; the numerous state government personnel who shared a mutual interest in our mission to serve children; and the connections with our state's five pediatric training programs at the time.

The relationships with the pediatric chairs at the medical schools—Sam Katz at Duke University, Floyd Denny at University of North Carolina, Jimmy Simon at Wake Forest University, Jon Tingelstad at East Carolina University, plus J.C. Parke of the pediatric department at then Charlotte Memorial Hospital—were of paramount importance. Not only were medical students and residents exposed to the value of joining the state pediatric organization, but the attention given to developments in clinical pediatric medicine and its importance for—and translation to—community practice helped contribute to NCPeds' growth. Pediatric department chairs were supportive of our efforts and helped to revitalize our efforts in difficult situations.

All of these efforts contributed to a heightened interest from pediatricians, and NCPeds' membership soared in numbers. In 1969, a printed roster showed a membership of 245 pediatricians. According to the treasurer's report for 1977, our membership was 300 pediatricians. The minutes of the September 1982 executive committee meeting reported a membership of 503 pediatricians. By 2008, we had

The Annual Meeting became a fixture
of NCPeds and a prime attraction that drew
members to an educational and social event.

gained an additional 800 new members for a total of 1,300 members. From the 1980s to the present, at the Academy level, North Carolina went from being a "medium" to a "large" to a "very large" chapter in membership. In 2023, NCPeds is one of the ten largest state pediatric organizations in North America, which includes Canada.

The loyalty to our annual meetings was strongly influenced by the pediatric departments, as many of the lectures and workshops featured faculty members. This is rooted in an annual event hosted by the dean of the Duke Medical School and founding organizer, Dr. Wilburt C. Davison, that began in the 1930s at his summer home in Roaring Gap, North Carolina. The annual meetings became a fixture of NCPeds and a prime attraction that drew members to an educational and social event. Attendance grew as membership increased, and the annual meeting remains a highlight on the annual calendar of activities. Member evaluations have consistently shown that the medical education, practice management, and child health advocacy topics are always timely, and the social events are well received by our members. The growth in attendance at the annual meeting matched our growth in membership.

There are few records of the membership files during the first two decades of NCPeds' existence. Most of the information gleaned comes from notations in the meeting minutes from the executive committee, as the original governing body of NCPeds was called. In addition, there is a file of membership applications for the years 1948–1997 that is a good secondary source of information about the application procedure and recognition of members. It has been discovered in this membership file that the society initiated yearly compulsory dues of five dollars ($5) per member in 1946. This procedural action by NCPeds is recorded by then Secretary-Treasurer Susan C. Dees of Durham in a 1948 letter of correspondence to a delinquent member. Dr. Dees was president in 1960.

From the founding of NCPeds in 1931, North Carolina created a unique condition that included doctors serving children, along with members who were Fellows in the Academy. This dual membership status worked harmoniously, and NCPeds took the organizational lead in planning the annual meeting, as well as a schedule of meetings for the executive committee to discuss the business of pediatrics in the state. NCPeds would meet at least once per year in conjunction with the NC Medical Society.

In most years this occurred at the famous Carolina Hotel in Pinehurst, which helped attract attendance. In 1974, the society and the chapter merged administrative operations to become one membership organization as the NC Chapter of the AAP, but retained the use of the name NC Pediatric Society, as the organization was originally founded and widely known around the state. Following a strategic planning exercise that culminated in 2013, the organization adopted the shortened NCPeds name for publications and brand identification.

In the decades before the chapter hired an executive director and administrative staff, membership records were kept on paper and note cards by the secretary-treasurer of the organization. I recall that James Rouse of Durham was treasurer when I was president, and we worked with Mrs. John McLain of Durham, who acted as executive secretary from 1960–1980, keeping the records of membership. She maintained a card file with the names of members—paid and not paid—and also assisted with dues collection and correspondence. The secretary-treasurer's position was divided into two separate offices with the election of new officers in 1975. During these years, many pediatric practice managers and clerical staff assisted the treasurer to keep track of members and dues. North Carolina had always encouraged not only pediatricians but any doctor who cared for children to join NCPeds. Membership in the American Academy of Pediatrics was not the focus of our membership efforts for much of this time. The NC Chapter of the AAP was formally recognized by the academy in 1956.

In 1979, designated as the International Year of the Child by the United Nations, Governor James B. Hunt Jr. signed a comprehensive "Child Health Plan for Raising a New Generation," developed by many participants in state government with the participation of twenty-three pediatricians. This remarkable effort was co-chaired by Thomas Frothingham, MD, FAAP, of Duke Medical School and myself as president of NCPeds. Unfortunately, upon its completion, the overall plan languished without state appropriations and no further investment of political capital or even legislative interest. In spite of that, many of the specific priorities in the plan were diligently achieved because they provided practical guidance for pediatricians who stepped into the spotlight of child advocacy across North Carolina.

Beginning in the early 1980s and lasting until 1998, several NC Medical Society staff members assisted NCPeds with administration and meeting planning, including Carolyn Russell, Patrick Kennedy, and Alan Skipper. These were dedicated staff who served the organization with commendation. This arrangement was satisfactory until our organization registered enough members to hire an executive director and other staff to manage our affairs.

There was one special circumstance at this time that proved instrumental in helping generate interest in NCPeds: our interdependence with the NC Medicaid program, called the Division of Medical Assistance, in state government parlance, led by Director Barbara Matula. Matula was a staunch child health advocate and wanted North Carolina physicians to increase their participation in Medicaid; however, the gap in fees paid by Medicaid versus private health insurance and Medicare fees was a barrier and proved to be a financial hardship for many practices with a high number of Medicaid patients. The pressure to negotiate higher fees intensified when Dr. David T. Tayloe Sr. succeeded me to become chapter president for 1982–84. Dr. Sarah Morrow, secretary of the NC Department of Human Resources (recently reorganized as the Department of Health and Human Services) under Governor Hunt, supported efforts to increase Medicaid payments. Dr. Tayloe Sr. made increasing the Medicaid fee schedule a focus of his term as president.

The slow and steady improvement in the fees paid by Medicaid for pediatric care was a boost for every medical practice that served Medicaid patients, and helped many pediatricians recognize the value of membership in NCPeds. Matula's attendance at the NCPeds liaison committee meetings in North Carolina and her appearances at the governmental affairs committee at the national meetings of the American Academy of Pediatrics helped to highlight the strong connections with state government that were being built and encouraged in North Carolina. I have always maintained that pediatricians' first interest was in the children, and all of the efforts to increase payment were primarily so pediatric offices could remain viable and continue to deliver quality care to our patients.

At the conclusion of my term as president, I made the decision to chair the membership committee. I took a personal approach to the effort to retain our existing members and to work at recruiting new members. Many pediatricians across the state who were already members assisted me when I made contact with them about partners or other pediatric practices in their town or county, as well as surrounding communities.

I can cite quite a few pediatricians who, like me, made personal contacts, inviting and coaxing either partners or practicing pediatricians who were acquaintances in the area. These include Doctors: Norman Parks in Asheville; Bill Horn in Boone; Carolyn Cort in Burnsville; David Dyer in Waynesville; Fletcher Raiford and Mike Dennis in Hendersonville; James Thomas in Morganton; Curtis Abell in Statesville; Jerry Froedge in Hickory; Tom Carlton Jr. in Salisbury; Lee Gilliatt in Shelby; Jerry Marder and George Prince in Gastonia; Henry Johnson in Winston-Salem; Paige Follo and James Singer in Greensboro; Charlie Scott in Burlington; James Rouse in Durham; Charlie Shaffer in Chapel Hill; J.C. Parke, Henry Smith and Griggs Dickson in Charlotte; George Engstrom in Concord; Jim McQueen and Jim Smithwick in Laurinburg; Elwood Coley, Bob Young and Thad Wester in Lumberton; Archie Johnson and Bill Hubbard in Raleigh; Dave Tayloe Jr. in Goldsboro; Mac Herring in

Clinton; Tom Irons in Greenville; Dave Tayloe Sr., who made contacts in a lot of towns in eastern NC including Kinston, New Bern and Rocky Mount from his location in Washington; George Hemingway in Tarboro; Dick Kelley, Tom McCutcheon and Pierre LeMaster in Fayetteville; and Charlie Hicks, Frank Reynolds, Gordon Coleman and Henry Hawthorne in Wilmington.

This is but a sample of the pediatricians across North Carolina who helped to grow the membership of NCPeds by making personal calls and contacts. Aside from the quarterly newsletter, there was not much mail from the executive committee to the members during the year, but the liaison committee meetings that moved around the state and the annual meeting provided a framework for recruiting and retaining members once they were approved for membership.

As computers came into use in the late 1990s, the American Academy of Pediatrics converted from sending paper records by mail to the state membership chairs to using email to send records to either the membership chair or to the NCPeds office. North Carolina had established its own office in 1998 with Dave Rock as the executive director. He hired administrative assistant Petra Harris to assist me in reviewing the computer-generated list of members who were current on dues and those who needed to be reminded to pay dues. Rock also did NCPeds a "forever favor" when he created the first spreadsheet of members based on the academy's records so we could always compare our own trusted membership file with the academy's roster to make sure no member was lost in the conversion from paper to computer records.

When Steve Shore became the full-time executive director, he hired administrative assistants Amelia McDaniels Johnson, Diane Lewis Sloane, Megan Coward Gaines, Jennifer Wheeler, John Meidl, and Kim Day, CPA, respectively during the years 1999–2014. Each of these staff members assisted me by managing our in-house database of membership and interpreting the monthly roster from the American Academy of Pediatrics for each category of membership. This allowed me to continue the practice of making personal contacts and using members to encourage partners and other local pediatricians to consider joining NCPeds.

NCPeds did not charge a membership fee to medical students or residents, thereby encouraging their participation during their years of training. Member dues were charged only to fellows, associates and several categories of affiliates, including child and adolescent psychiatrists, pediatric dentists and fellows from out of state who wanted to maintain membership in NCPeds. In the 1990s, NCPeds opened associate membership to practice managers, social workers, psychologists, physician assistants and nurse practitioners, which allowed our administrative and allied health personnel to participate in chapter affairs to improve business practice and clinical care.

When President Jane Foy, MD, called for the organization of a practice managers section in 1998, no one could have predicted the group's impact. Dave Rock, executive director from 1998–99, set up the first meeting. The practice managers section became one of the most effective and productive work groups, promoting a successful primary care business model and capitalizing on the notion of a medical home for children. In 2003, NCPeds established the first member listserv and our managers worked together to assure that every practice could share in problem solving that ranged from billing and coding to vaccine supply and storage to waste management contracting. In some years, the group conducted salary and benefit surveys to gauge how pediatric practices compared to other primary care providers.

In several years during my term as membership chair, the academy recognized North Carolina for having 100 percent annual retention of members. I am proud of this, but it shows how our organization valued teamwork in promoting our activities, our advocacy agenda, and staging the annual meetings. I hope these notes illustrate how North Carolina nurtured a sense of community and collaboration in everything that NCPeds conducted. It helps explain the success of our organization in attracting and retaining pediatrician members over the years.

## Immunizations: Essential Component of the Pediatric Medical Home

by Beth Rowe-West, RN, BSN; Dave Tayloe Jr., MD, FAAP

In 1982, there was a disturbing documentary telecast on national network television depicting eleven young children in Great Britain who were thought to have suffered severe brain damage from the whooping cough vaccine[1]. Almost overnight, there were lawsuits brought against physicians and vaccine manufacturers concerning US children who may have suffered similar vaccine-related injury.

David Tayloe Sr., MD, FAAP, president of NCPeds from 1981–83, became the target of one of these lawsuits, being found negligent or legally responsible during a jury trial in 1985. This led to NCPeds working to convince the NC General Assembly to successfully pass epic tort reform legislation in 1986 to protect physicians and vaccine manufacturers from jury trials in medical malpractice cases involving state-mandated vaccines. (see *Big Dave: Visionary Leader*)

This vaccine liability crisis caused vaccine prices to skyrocket. Physicians bought diphtheria-tetanus-pertussis (DTaP) vaccines for only fifteen cents per dose in 1980, but by 1990, the price was about ten dollars per dose! Physicians were sending unimmunized children out of their offices to local health departments to receive free

---

[1] It took scientists until 2006 to identify a genetic disease, Dravet Syndrome, that accounted for 9 of the 11 patients' neurological symptoms.

state vaccines because of these price increases. In 1987, at the insistence of President Bob Schwartz, MD, FAAP, NCPeds began working to convince state leaders to create a universal vaccine program for North Carolina, whereby the state would buy all the vaccines needed for all eligible children and distribute those vaccines to all physicians who wished to participate in the universal program. The estimated cost in 1987 was $2.5 million dollars. During this time, NCPeds developed a very productive relationship with the administrators in the immunization branch of NC state government and began working to solve the escalating problems in the childhood immunization arena.

The universal vaccine program proposal could not get traction until David Bruton, MD, convinced newly elected Governor Jim Hunt to put $16 million dollars into his 1994 budget proposal to fund a universal childhood vaccine program. In 1993, the federal government created the Vaccines for Children Program (VFC). This would give money to states to provide free vaccines for all children who were eligible for Medicaid, uninsured, underinsured, Native American, or American Eskimo. This federal program allowed Governor Hunt to reduce his proposed appropriation to $8 million dollars. The federal government also created a table of allowable vaccine administration fees to be paid by Medicaid, or charged to other patients, so that providers could recover their administrative costs for participating in the childhood immunization program. NCPeds negotiated the maximum allowable immunization administration fee for participating providers in North Carolina.

In 1994, the NC General Assembly appropriated funding to enhance vaccine availability for children not covered by a program of the Centers for Disease Control (CDC): VFC to create what became known as the North Carolina Universal Childhood Vaccine Distribution Program (UCVDP). In large part, the creation of this program was due to the advocacy of NCPeds.

The CDC's National Immunization Survey reported an estimated vaccine coverage rate of 58 percent for North Carolina's two-year-old children prior to the introduction of the UCVDP. By 2001, the state's immunization coverage rates led the nation with a rate of 88 percent for that same age group.

Although state and national funding were critical to develop the infrastructure necessary to make such massive improvements in coverage rates, much of the success is attributed to the partnership of the UCVDP and NCPeds. At the peak of enrollment, approximately 96 percent of North Carolina's pediatricians were participating in the UCVDP program, administering over 75 percent of childhood vaccines in the children's medical homes. This meant children could be vaccinated in their medical homes without the missed opportunities that occurred previously.

The relationship of this partnership between public health and NCPeds remained strong throughout the existence of the UCVDP. NCPeds championed the program

Although state and national funding were critical to develop the infrastructure necessary to make such massive improvements in coverage rates, much of the success is attributed to the partnership of the UCVDP and NCPeds.

from the beginning, contributing through advocacy and policy development. NCPeds' leadership often reached out to the UCVDP's leadership for one-on-one discussions whenever challenges arose. NCPeds invited the chief of the immunization branch to speak at all quarterly and annual meetings. There, at the meeting's Open Form, an open exchange of ideas occurred. This ultimately improved service delivery to children throughout the state, and frequently solved problems to meet state and federal requirements without jeopardizing the strength of services to children. North Carolina was the only state that could boast such a relationship. In fact, I was often asked, "How did you make this happen?" In actuality, it was the realization by leadership from both NCPeds and UCVDP that children would be best served with this exchange of ideas that resulted in improvements in the health of North Carolina's children.

In addition, the immunization branch formed the NC Immunization Advisory Committee (IAC) in 1997 to convene a panel of experts to advise the branch on a variety of immunization issues. The IAC was composed of representatives from school health, local public health, legal affairs, family medicine, and pediatrics. NCPeds sent the largest group, with seven pediatricians serving on the committee from its inception. The most senior member was Dr. Samuel Katz, chairman of the Department of Pediatrics at Duke University and a well-respected researcher and leader in the field of immunizations at the national and international levels. Dr. Katz is best known as a co-developer of the first measles vaccine. The immunization branch presented a bi-annual Dr. Sam Katz Award to a health professional making contributions to advance immunization services in his/her community. Topics for discussion by the IAC included appropriate minimal intervals for required vaccines, proper vaccine storage, and the selection of vaccines when multiple comparable products were available.

In 2013, NCPeds amended their board structure to include at-large members. This meant relationships with non-physician partners could further strengthen the work of the organization in meeting the needs of the children. Retiring as branch head in 2013, Beth Rowe-West was honored to become a member of this first reconfigured board. She served two terms and contributed to discussions that involved our state's immunization issues, national public health policies and trends, and information concerning other state jurisdictions.

Ms. Rowe-West commented, "It was a privilege to serve on the board of an organization willing to take the chance to include those outside their membership. I can only hope this structure continues to strengthen the high quality of services for North Carolina's children."

## Stepping Up Our Advocacy: Hiring an Experienced Lobbyist

by Henry W. Jones Jr., JD; Dave Tayloe Jr., MD, FAAP

Henry Jones Jr. began practicing law in Raleigh in 1978. On reflection, he stated, "I quickly developed an interest in representation of existing law firm clients before the NC General Assembly, beginning in 1979." Two of his earliest clients were healthcare-related organizations: NC Public Health Association and NC Veterinary Association. As a result of his work for these groups, a public health pediatrician Dr. Jimmie Rhyne recommended Jones for the NCPeds' lobbyist position.

Dr. Steve Edwards of Raleigh contacted Jones, asked for a proposal, and requested a personal meeting. That interview was conducted at Edwards' office where he explained NCPeds' budget and general legislative goals. We met for about an hour, and also indicated that Jones was competing for the position with a former governor, which Jones later recalled was "a bit daunting for a 28-year-old lobbyist, but I remained optimistic that I would get the engagement. NCPeds did decide to hire me on a year-to-year basis, and I began to lobby for the society during the general session in 1983."

### EARLY EFFORTS

NCPeds had a deep interest in obtaining more funding for the state's Perinatal and Crippled Children's programs. "I always remember Dr. Jimmy Simon, chairperson of the Department of Pediatrics at the Wake Forest University School of Medicine and both a leader in NCPeds and in these efforts to secure funding for these children's programs," said Jones. With Dr. Simon's motivation, the lobbying efforts were rewarded with special funding during these years to support the programs, even though state budgets were tight and such appropriations were hard to secure. Fortunately, Lieutenant Governor Jimmy Green was a major supporter of these programs and was instrumental in helping us obtain needed appropriations during the early years.

## SAFETY LEGISLATION

By attending every executive committee and liaison committee meeting in 1983 and 1984, Jones became better acquainted with the members of NCPeds and learned more about their needs and agendas. Safety legislation became a very important part of NCPeds' agenda. The passage of NC Child Restraint Legislation was highly significant because it became the second such state-mandated legislation in the US.

**Comments from Mike Lawless, MD, FAAP:** Being a part of the effort by our NC Chapter of the AAP to seek child passenger safety legislation in North Carolina introduced me to the importance of advocacy for children beyond providing for their medical care. While child safety car seats were developed in the mid-1970s, the first law requiring restraint of child passengers was passed by Tennessee in 1978. In 1979, NCPeds formed a Transportation Safety Committee, which I chaired for several years. We sought similar legislation to protect North Carolina's child passengers. Our committee worked in concert with the NC Governor's Highway Safety Program and other advocacy groups. It took several years of lobbying and educating our lawmakers to achieve our goal. The first law enacted by our legislature was disappointing because it had exceptions, such as allowing a mother to travel with her unprotected baby in her arms if she was breastfeeding the infant. Child safety advocates called this exception "the child-crusher amendment." It took additional years to gradually strengthen the law both by removing exceptions and by expanding the age of children who should be restrained. In 1981, the "First Ride ... A Safe Ride" program established by the American Academy of Pediatrics served as an additional resource for education and advocacy for child passenger safety.

> The passage of the NC Child Restraint Legislation was highly significant because it became the second such state-mandated legislation in the country.

Valuable child advocacy lessons learned from this experience included the importance of: embracing other like-minded partners in order to strengthen one's advocacy voice; employing a lobbyist to maximize influence and outreach to legislators; recruiting one or more members of the legislature to be a champion for

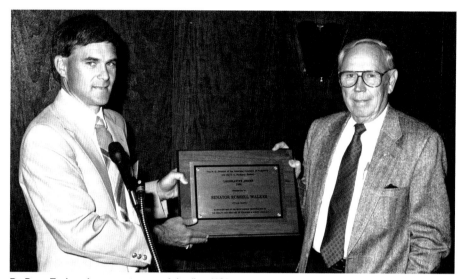

**Dr. Dave Tayloe, Jr. presents one of the first NCPeds awards to Senator Russell Walker in 1988.**

our cause; realizing that while our initial attempt(s) to pass proposed legislation may be unsuccessful, getting even a weak version of a hoped-for law is a start; and lastly, recognizing that the initial law can be improved by continued efforts.

Pediatricians who participated in this important initiative made good use of the lessons learned in future advocacy endeavors, such as supporting legislation that required the wearing of bike helmets. The individual pediatrician, in practice, has a key role in educating families about proper use of car seats and seat belts. It is rewarding to think of how many young lives have been saved by legislation requiring effective child passenger safety.

That success led to the effort to pass legislation regulating water heater temperatures in order to prevent burns on small children.

**Comments by Dave Tayloe Jr., MD, FAAP:** Hot water coming from home water heaters is a cause of frequent, significant, thermal injury for children. Home water heaters should be set at 120°F or less if children are to be protected from thermal injury. During the 1980s, based upon model AAP state legislation, NCPeds attempted to pass legislation to require homebuilders to set water heaters at 120°F or less in all new construction. It took three different campaigns in three different sessions of the General Assembly to achieve success. Henry Jones, as the lobbyist for NCPeds, deserves all the credit for persevering until this important child safety issue could be successfully addressed by the legislature.

For a description of the water heater statute, see *Appendix: Legislation Referenced in Commentary by Jones and Tayloe.*

## CHILD FATALITY TASK FORCE

In 1990, NCPeds and leaders like John Niblock, executive director of the NC Child Advocacy Institute, urged the General Assembly to create an official standing legislative study commission, which became known as the NC Child Fatality Task Force. The task force gave stakeholders a forum to vet various child safety ideas and to ease the bill introduction process in the General Assembly. In reality, over the ensuing decades, the Child Fatality Task Force became a strategic think tank and incubator for a variety of important legislative issues affecting children and families.

## GUN RESPONSIBILITY LEGISLATION

With that success, NCPeds decided to take on gun responsibility legislation. The gun legislation was highly controversial, but it put NCPeds at the forefront of child safety and brought a great amount of public exposure. North Carolina was still politically and culturally a conservative state, and this legislation tested the limits of the legislature's willingness to regulate behavior on behalf of children in the state. Through this legislation, which was enacted in 1993, it enabled and strengthened our work to single out and identify child advocates in the legislature who were willing to push the limits and speak out with great force on behalf of children and child safety.

**Comments by Dave Tayloe Jr., MD, FAAP:** In 1993, NCPeds reviewed legislation passed in Florida and Maine that allowed the states to prosecute gun owners whose guns were used by minors to inflict injury on themselves or others. As chair of our committee on legislation, I worked with Henry Jones Jr., JD, lobbyist for the chapter, to have a similar bill introduced into our legislative session. Henry linked me with Greg Malhoit, a Raleigh-based consultant who seemed to know how it might be possible to convince the General Assembly leadership to pass such legislation. Mr. Jones and I met with Mr. Malhoit at Big Ed's Restaurant in downtown Raleigh one morning to formulate a strategy that resulted in a big win for children.

For details on the gun responsibility legislation, see *Appendix: Legislation Referenced in Commentary by Jones and Tayloe.*

## PICKUP TRUCK BILL

NCPeds was gaining confidence in passing legislative agenda. In 1994, NCPeds lobbied for the so-called "Pickup Truck Bill" that limited the ability of people to carry children less than twelve years old in the open bed of a pickup truck. Regulating the use of pickup trucks tested the limits of safety regulation and the will of the General

Assembly, for sure. Jones remembers the statement made by the late Senator John Kerr of Wayne County, who, while a supporter of the legislation, warned: "This is about as far as I think we can go in regulating safety in North Carolina."

**Comments from Dave Tayloe Jr., MD, FAAP:** In the 1990s, the American Academy of Pediatrics promoted state legislation that would prohibit minors from riding in the backs of pickup trucks. As chair of the NCPeds Committee on Legislation, I worked with Representative Carolyn Russell (R-Wayne), my local representative, to introduce this bill into the General Assembly in 1995, and Representative Russell was able to convince the House to pass the bill. The bill, as referred to the Senate, would prohibit children under the age of twelve years from riding in the back of a pickup truck unless there was an adult riding in the back of the truck with the children.

There was strong support for the bill in the Senate, but the chair of the Judicial Committee to whom the bill was referred for mark-up was Frank Ballance, a lawyer from a very rural northeastern county. Senator Ballance was opposed to the bill because he believed that many low-income residents in his county had no way to transport their children if they could not allow them to ride in the backs of pickup trucks. Senator Balance refused to bring the bill to a vote in the committee as the session wound down toward adjournment.

To complain about the fact that this very important child safety measure was being held hostage by Senator Balance, when it would probably pass if the senator would bring the bill to a vote in committee, I called the office of Senator Marc Basnight, president pro tempore of the Senate, and a rural eastern North Carolina friend who went to church with my mother-in-law. I was seeing patients in our pediatric practice that day and was unable to talk with Senator Basnight, but did have a phone conversation with a member of the Senator's staff. I explained to the staff member that Senator Ballance was being very stubborn in his opposition to this "motherhood and apple pie" children's legislation, and that Senator Basnight needed to firmly insist that Senator Ballance bring the bill to a vote in the committee.

Shortly after that conversation, my nurse informed me that I needed to take an incoming call from Senator Basnight. The senator asked me why I had been so critical of Senator Balance, and I responded by explaining to Senator Basnight that this important bill needed to pass before adjournment of the session, and that the bill would pass if Senator Ballance would allow the committee to vote on the bill. Senator Basnight then contacted Senator Ballance about the need to allow the committee to vote on the bill. Senator Ballance did allow the committee to vote on the bill, but successfully had it amended to exclude from the legislation counties with fewer than 3,500 people.

The bill then was passed in the committee and later on the floor of the Senate, thus becoming law. Since 1995, the law has been amended to include children under the age of sixteen, and to get rid of the exemption for any counties. It does exempt agricultural enterprises, use for emergencies, and parades.

In 1990, NCPeds, along with such leaders as John Niblock of NC Child Advocacy Institute, urged the North Carolina General Assembly to create a standing study commission which became known as the NC Child Fatality Study Task Force, which gave stakeholders a forum to introduce and vet various child safety ideas and to ease the introduction process in the General Assembly. In reality, the NC Child Fatality Study Task Force became a think tank and incubator for a variety of important legislative issues affecting children and families.

## VACCINE INJURY LEGISLATION

From 1985-1986, Dave Tayloe Jr., Henry Jones Jr., and a large representation of NCPeds members helped create a movement in North Carolina that was instrumental in addressing a catastrophic vaccine injury liability judgment that resulted in the first of its kind legislation in the nation. (see *Big Dave: Visionary Leader*)

## HENRY W. JONES, JR., JD REFLECTS ON WORKING WITH NCPEDS

The NCPeds legislative program was, in my opinion, remarkably successful. The leadership was uniformly dynamic and excellent. The liaison committee was composed of pediatricians and health care advocates in state government, academia, and private practice.

All of the greatest ideas and concepts were discussed and debated in that diverse committee. The executive committee made the final decisions on behalf of NCPeds and gave me, as lobbyist, my marching orders. The executive committee was composed of knowledgeable, dedicated practitioners who were very practical and always decisive. I never had a question about my agenda, and I was always given the support and resources needed to do my best on behalf of the society.

Dave Tayloe Jr. and I liked to make the rounds in the NC General Assembly. He would call me when he had hours to spare, travel to Raleigh, meet me, and walk around the NC General Assembly to make contact with key legislators on issues of interest, or I would just update him on major pending legislation.

We had some very effective sessions in Raleigh, particularly during those person-to-person contacts. By 1987, Dr. Tayloe was known throughout the state and had instant visibility and credibility. He was an incredible advocate for children's health in North Carolina and the two of us made a very good team as we made our rounds in Raleigh.

# Whys and Hows of Medicaid

**by Tork Wade, MPH**

While North Carolina is widely recognized for its innovative statewide medical home and care management system, the reality is that Community Care of North Carolina (CCNC) did not rise up as a finished vision; rather, it evolved over thirty years, adapting to changing needs and constantly refining its approach. Along every step of this evolution, North Carolina pediatricians played critical roles.

## CREATION OF CAROLINA ACCESS (1989–97)

The first major step in this evolution was the formation of the Carolina Access Program. In 1989, under the leadership of Jim Bernstein, director of the NC Office of Rural Health, and Barbara Matula, North Carolina Medicaid director, North Carolina began rolling out this basic medical home program that linked North Carolina Medicaid children and mothers to participating primary care physicians across the state. For a small three-dollar-per-member-per-month (PMPM) care-coordination fee, physicians agreed to provide and coordinate enrollees' care.

By the end of 1997, Carolina Access was in place in ninety-nine out of 100 North Carolina counties with 2,000 participating primary care physicians. Mecklenburg County, with 650,000 Medicaid beneficiaries and North Carolina's most populous county, was a private insurance plan health maintenance organization (HMO) county that later became a Carolina Access county when an evaluation of the HMO program showed much poorer performance than the networks under physician-directed Carolina Access.

The program achieved its primary goal of providing seventy percent of Medicaid women and children with a medical home and in decreasing non-emergent use of hospital emergency departments by more than thirty percent.

While many pediatricians played pivotal roles in the successful rollout of the Carolina Access Program, NCPeds leaders were essential. During the rollout period, Doctors Robert Schwartz, Stephen Edwards, Dave Tayloe Jr. (Dr. Tayloe currently serves as a Community Care of North Carolina board member), and Olson Huff served as NCPeds Presidents and were, along with the society's Executive Director, Steve Shore, indispensable in achieving great participation by pediatricians across the state. This North Carolina Pediatric Society/Medicaid partnership proved to be a key to North Carolina developing the most innovative Medicaid program in the country.

**EARLY DAYS OF COMMUNITY CARE OF NORTH CAROLINA (1997–2001),
MOVING TO A NEW SYSTEM**

In the mid-1990s, the federal government shifted more of the financial and administrative responsibility for Medicaid to the states. With this looming prospect, the secretary of the NC Department of Health and Human Services (NC DHHS), and founder of Sandhills Pediatrics in Moore County, pediatrician David Bruton, MD, wanted to build on Carolina Access to create the next-generation Medicaid program that could deliver better budget predictability. The new program would strengthen the Carolina Access medical home by introducing four new supports to enhance the ability of primary care physicians to improve patient care and outcomes:

- **The Formation of Networks**

  Physicians would be encouraged to work together locally and with other key community health organizations in delivering care. The focus would be on recipients with chronic conditions.

- **Introduction of Population Management Tools**

  To arm physicians and practices with tools needed to improve care outcomes, the new program would introduce physician-designed evidence-based protocols, disease management programs, practice-based improvements, and pharmacy management tools.

- **Care Management**

  The new program would also provide physicians and patients with the care management support needed to help patients that have complex medical, social, and behavioral health conditions manage their care.

- **Data and Feedback**

  Because participating physicians had very limited information about patient progress and outcomes, the new program would focus on providing timely and relevant information about how patients and interventions were progressing and would identify opportunities for improvement.

Under the new program, Carolina Access practices were given two options. They could work together as physician practices and form a horizontal network that would cross many communities, or they could collaborate with other local practices and health organizations to form a community network.

Twenty-six practices, almost all of them pediatric, elected to form a statewide physician network known as AccessCare. Joe Ponzi MD, FAAP (who had been medical director for Carolina Access), a pediatric leader from Goldsboro, would serve as board chair, and Steve Wegner, JD, MD, FAAP, a pediatrician who had practiced in Dunn, North Carolina, would become president. Other key AccessCare pediatrician leaders who served on the board were: Doctors Dave Williams, Debbie Ainsworth, Alan Stiles, and Stephen Edwards.

Nine practices wanted to form community networks. Once again, pediatric leaders were pivotal in forming these networks. Doctors Susan Mims, president of NCPeds for 2018-2020 and Olson Huff in the Buncombe County region, Chuck Willson and Tom Irons in the Pitt County region, Jane Foy in the Forsyth County region, Dennis Clements in the Durham County region, Betsey Tilson in the Wake County region, Marion Earls in the Guilford County region (Dr. Earls also later served as director of Pediatric Programs for Community Care), and David Bruton and Bill Stewart in the Sandhills region. During these significant development efforts, Senator Bill Purcell, pediatrician founder of the Purcell Clinic in Laurinburg, North Carolina, was a key legislative leader in securing legislative support for these Medicaid innovations.

## COMMUNITY CARE OF NORTH CAROLINA BECOMES A STATEWIDE PROGRAM (2001–21)

Under the leadership of NC DHHS Secretary Carmen Hooker Odom and Assistant Secretary of Health and Medicaid Director Dr. Allen Dobson, Community Care, which had achieved excellent results in managing the Aid to Families with Dependent Children (AFDC), was asked to begin managing the costliest Medicaid recipients, the aged, blind and disabled (ABD) populations. To accomplish this, Community Care would reorganize to become a system of local networks.

By 2011, Community Care included fourteen networks that covered all 100 counties and served more than 1.5 million Medicaid beneficiaries as well as 70,000 low-income uninsured residents through the HealthNet[2] program.

These efforts have improved the quality of patient care and saved the state millions of dollars each year, as calculated by outside actuaries. In 2010, Milliman, Inc. estimated total program savings of $984 million over a four-year period.

In 2007, The John F. Kennedy School of Government at Harvard University and the Annie E. Casey Foundation awarded Community Care the Innovations Award in Children and Family Service. CCNC also received the Hearst Prize for Innovation in Population Health. The extensive and effective participation of North Carolina pediatricians in Community Care was a key reason the state received these awards.

---

[2] HealthNet was established in 2005 by the NC General Assembly to connect safety net organizations (such as free clinics, public health departments, school-based clinics) to Community Care of North Carolina networks to provide low-income, uninsured residents with a medical home and access to prescription drugs and care coordination. Grant funds covered infrastructure costs. The Office of Rural Health (ORH) was providing more than $4 million annually to CCNC networks and partners. At its peak, Health Net was annually connecting low-income, uninsured residents to more than 32,000 medical homes and providing care management to 26,000 individuals. The value of donated physician services exceeded more than $10 million annually. The program ended on June 30, 2015.

**COMMUNITY CARE IN NORTH CAROLINA'S TRANSITION TO MANAGED CARE**

In 2015, North Carolina began preparations to shift to a statewide managed care system for Medicaid. This major shift proved to be a catalyst for significant changes in Community Care:

- To be able to effectively contract with the new Prepaid Health Plans (PHPs) (five plans won State contracts), CCNC moved from a system of fourteen independent networks to a single central organization that had the capability to contract with PHPs and to deliver outstanding results in the areas of access, quality, and cost-effectiveness. CCNC was able to secure significant contracts with all five of the PHPs.
- To succeed under the new system change, CCNC would restructure its core business by standardizing and streamlining care management and practice support and developing new analytical tools. A seamless infrastructure is now in place across North Carolina.
- In 2016, at the encouragement of the NC Pediatric Society, the NC Academy of Family Physicians, and the NC Community Health Center Association, Community Care partnered with its independent primary care physicians to launch the Community Care Physician Network (CCPN), LLC, a clinically integrated network of 3,200 independent primary care clinicians in 930 practices. Such pediatric leaders as Drs. Beverly Edwards, Christoph Diasio, Greg Adams (who also serves as a CCPN co-president), and Larry Mann are CCPN board members, and Graham Barden serves on the contract committee. Through CCPN, member physicians have contracts with all five participating PHPs and seven other payor contracts (Medicare-based).

The new system went live on July 1, 2021. The transition was extremely smooth because of real-time communication involving physicians, CCNC staff, key Medicaid administrators, and PHP leaders.

# School-Based Hepatitis B Immunization

**by Dave Tayloe Jr., MD, FAAP**

I met Sam Katz, MD, FAAP, at an annual meeting of NCPeds in the late 1970s at the Blockade Runner Hotel in Wrightsville Beach, North Carolina. At that time, Sam was the chairman of the department of pediatrics at Duke University. He came to Duke from Boston, where he had worked with the inventors of the measles vaccine. I also met his wife, Catherine Wilfert, MD, FAAP, an eminent pediatric infectious diseases subspecialist who later blazed trails in preventing the perinatal transmission of HIV.

My dad, president-elect of the society at the time, introduced me to Sam and Cathy while he was trying to teach them to body surf in the ocean in front of the hotel. Sam lost a very nice pair of sunglasses during that memorable experience!

My relationship with Sam grew during the 1980s when he helped me convince the NC General Assembly that we needed tort reform legislation to protect physicians from frivolous vaccine-injury lawsuits. I also called Sam from time to time to obtain consultation on challenging infectious disease problems in our practice.

In 1991, the Advisory Committee on Immunization Practice (ACIP) at the Centers for Disease Control (CDC) recommended that all children receive a three-dose series of the hepatitis B vaccine and that the first dose be given as soon after birth as possible. Many pediatricians thought we should be able to give the vaccine to older children because much of the morbidity and mortality of hepatitis B occurs in adolescents and young adults secondary to unsafe sexual activity and intravenous drug use. I called Dr. Katz to ask why the vaccine was not recommended for older children and why we could not give the vaccine to eligible children in our schools.

Dr. Katz did not think the healthcare system could reach adolescents to implement a vaccine program. However, newborns and infants were regularly in physicians' offices and health departments. I advised Sam that I was on a local board of education and worked closely with the schools and the health department and that we could give hepatitis B vaccines at school. Sam offered to find a grant for the NC Immunization Branch to pilot school-based hepatitis B immunization.

The federal authorities accepted the grant proposal, and the NC Immunization Branch selected health departments in Wayne (my home county) and Caldwell counties to pilot a fourth-grade hepatitis B immunization project. We immunized more than 70 percent of fourth graders in these two rural counties. After the pilot, the state implemented school-based hepatitis B immunization in the sixth grade for all 100 NC counties. This program was sunset when all the babies who began receiving the hepatitis B vaccine in 1991 reached at least the seventh grade.

NCPeds worked closely with the NC Immunization Branch to assure optimal pediatrician participation in the school-based immunization program. The immunization branch gave NCPeds' leadership regular updates on the program during the society's three yearly liaison committee/open forum meetings.

I am not sure our state would have become a leader in hepatitis B immunization if I had not become friends with Sam Katz during NCPeds meetings.

# Governor Jim Hunt and David Bruton, MD: Key Government Players for NCPeds

**by Dave Tayloe Jr., MD, FAAP**

During the 1980s, vaccine prices rose during the medical liability crisis along with concerns about the whooping cough (pertussis) vaccine safety. No insurance companies provided coverage for vaccine-related costs of physicians. NCPeds president for 1987-89, Bob Schwartz, MD, FAAP, encouraged Dave Tayloe Jr., MD, FAAP, chair of the chapter committee on legislation, to develop an appropriation request for the NC General Assembly so that the state could purchase all the vaccines for all the children of the state.

The Immunization Branch assisted Dr. Tayloe in developing an appropriation request for $2.5 million to establish a universal childhood vaccine program. This request did not gain traction in the state legislature until several years later when David Bruton, MD, convinced Governor Jim Hunt (1993–2001) to put an appropriation in the 1993–94 budget for $16 million to allow the Immunization Branch to purchase all recommended vaccines for all children; the price-tag increased from 1986 to 1993 because vaccine prices continued to rise, and hepatitis B and hemophilus influenzae type B vaccines were added to the other recommended vaccines (diphtheria-tetanus-pertussis, polio, and measles-mumps-rubella).

Dr. Bruton had a long-term relationship with Governor Hunt and was chosen by Governor Hunt to chair the state board of education (1977–82) and to be secretary of the NC Department of Health and Human Services (1997–2000). He practiced primary care pediatrics in Southern Pines, North Carolina. Under the leadership of Governor Hunt, the General Assembly established and funded the NC Universal Childhood Vaccine Distribution Program, assuring that all children would be able to receive all vaccines in all participating primary care settings.

Simultaneously, with strong encouragement from the American Academy of Pediatrics, the United States Congress established and funded the Vaccines for Children (VFC) Program whereby in 1993, the federal government agreed to pay for all vaccines for children in certain categories including Medicaid-eligible, uninsured, under-insured Native American, and American Eskimo. Under VFC, states were instructed to establish immunization administration fees that providers could charge patients to cover immunization-related costs of participating providers. Dr. Tayloe and Henry Smith, MD, FAAP, met with the Commission on Health Services and negotiated an agreement where Medicaid agreed to pay providers the maximum-allowed federal recommended fees for NC, $13.71, to administer the first vaccine and twenty-five dollars when two or more vaccines were given during a given practice encounter. This agreement was the first time providers had ever been paid separately by Medicaid for their immunization-related costs. Because of the federal VFC funding, Governor Hunt's recommended appropriation could be reduced to approximately $8 million per year.

Dr. Tayloe joined Governor Hunt in Raleigh to pack the first box of "free vaccines" to mail out to a primary care practice in North Carolina, and footage of this event appeared on the Raleigh evening news. Recalling these extraordinary events, Governor Hunt commented:

> With the increase in the number of recommended vaccines for children and rising prices of vaccines, we knew that many children would not be able to afford to pay for necessary vaccines unless the state stepped up and established and provided funding for the NC Universal Childhood Vaccine Distribution Program. I am proud to partner with the state's physicians, especially the NC Chapter of the American Academy of Pediatrics, in developing this most essential public health program.

In the years following the implementation of the universal vaccine program in NC, childhood immunization rates rose significantly to all-time high levels.

Congress established the Child Health Insurance Program (CHIP) within the Balanced Budget Act of 1997. Governor Hunt, with the assistance of Dr. Bruton, who served as secretary of Health and Human Services, quickly appointed a CHIP Task Force chaired by Tom Vitaglione, MPH, a friend of NCPeds and administrator in the division of maternal and child health services. Several pediatricians, including Olson Huff, MD, FAAP, and Dr. Dave Tayloe Jr. were appointed to this task force that met during the summer and fall of 1997 to develop a CHIP proposal for the 1998 General Assembly session. Governor Hunt called the General Assembly into a special session on March 24, 1998, to assure that our state could obtain the federal CHIP dollars to increase the number of low-income children who could receive comprehensive health services.

During this session, Mr. Vitaglione, Dr. Huff, and Dr. Tayloe led negotiations with Republican House and Democratic Senate leaders to develop a bipartisan CHIP proposal that the General Assembly approved. Even though the Republican-dominated House could not endorse recommendation of the Governor's Task Force's for a "Medicaid Look-alike" CHIP plan, the governor respected the opinions of the pediatrician leaders of the chapter. He signed the bill establishing NC Health Choice, a private insurance program administered by Blue Cross Blue Shield of NC. Governor Hunt appointed Wallace Brown, MD, FAAP, to chair the CHIP Oversight Committee and Dr. Dave Tayloe Jr. to chair the CHIP Committee on Children with Special Health Care Needs.

Recalling the political struggle during the CHIP Special Session of the General Assembly in 1998, Governor Hunt commented:

> I am disappointed that the NC General Assembly could not come together and endorse the CHIP plan put forward by Dr. Bruton and our Task Force and supported by the Senate. However, I am encouraged by the fact that the pediatricians were able to work with the House of Representatives leadership to develop an alternative plan that will give thousands of low-income children access to comprehensive health services comparable to those covered in Medicaid. We had to compromise on CHIP because we absolutely could not afford to allow the General Assembly to adjourn the special session without creating a CHIP plan whereby our state could receive maximum federal funding to serve as many low-income children as possible.

# Medicaid Crisis of 1996

**by Dave Tayloe Jr., MD, FAAP**

During the mid-nineties, Duke University Medical Center recruited twelve smaller hospitals to form a hospital consortium to become the management entity for North Carolina Medicaid. The consortium leadership hired a lobbyist and began convincing legislators and government administrators that the consortium could manage Medicaid better than a government agency.

After developing its strategy for obtaining legislative approval of the plan, the consortium recruited physicians to join the Physicians Advisory Group (PAG). Federal Medicaid statutes require states to have PAGs, but to my knowledge, our state had never formally established one. I was one of the pediatricians invited to join the PAG and learn about the consortium's plans to take over Medicaid.

Another pediatrician recruited to join the PAG was David Bruton, MD, of Southern Pines. Dr. Bruton was just getting used to his new role as secretary of Health and Human Services under Governor Jim Hunt. Dr. Bruton and I were friends from many years of seeing each other at NCPeds meetings and discussing issues related to our similar rural, independent pediatric group practices.

Dr. Bruton and I attended only two of the PAG meetings before we determined that the consortium was trying to turn Medicaid into a health maintenance organization (HMO) that would be directed by the hospitals. Our vision of the "proposed new Medicaid" was that the state would write a check to the consortium, and the consortium would make sure the state did not lose money on Medicaid. NCPeds had been working diligently with the current Medicaid Director Barbara Matula, MPH,

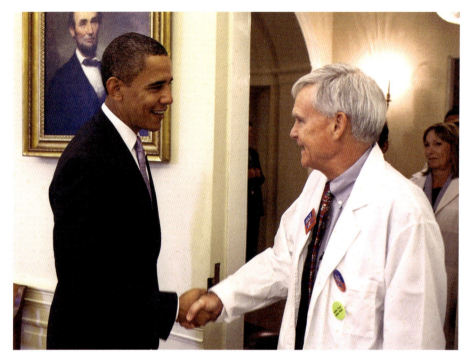

**President Barack Obama with Dave Tayloe Jr., MD, FAAP, AAP President**

and Director of the Office of Rural Health Jim Bernstein, to develop an innovative medical home program called Carolina Access (see *Whys and Hows of Medicaid*). Under Carolina Access, physician-directed boards would implement Medicaid in multiple networks, eventually covering the entire state. Dr. Bruton and I perceived the consortium plan to be contrary and adversarial to what was going on with the Carolina Access movement. Dr. Bruton and I resigned from the PAG and began doing what we could to defeat the legislative proposal of the consortium.

The NCPeds lobbyist could not help us because of conflicts with other clients relevant to health insurance issues. I worked within the NCPeds leadership as immediate past-president and chairperson of the committee on legislation to develop educational materials for members serving as key contacts for the 170 legislators in the NC General Assembly. Our key contact system consisted of thirteen House of Representatives coordinators and seven Senate coordinators. Each of the coordinators had five to ten key contact pediatricians that she/he was responsible for notifying about major legislative issues. I could make twenty calls to twenty pediatricians, and most of the General Assembly members would get a call from her/his local pediatrician. All this work was done by land-line telephone and "snail mail" before the days of online listservs, executive directors, and cell phones!

During this struggle, Barbara Matula resigned and retired as Medicaid director after an amazing seventeen-year tenure as our incredibly good friend and partner inside state government. We defeated the consortium proposal, thus preserving the opportunity to develop Carolina Access into Community Care of North Carolina, probably the premier Medicaid Program in the country!

The lobbyist for the consortium was John Bode, an attorney in Raleigh and husband of my good friend, Lucy Bode. Lucy and I worked together on the NC Child Advocacy Institute Board. Lucy also "worshipped" my father, Dave Tayloe Sr., MD, from their days serving together on the NC Medical Care Commission. John's brother, Bob, and I were fraternity brothers at UNC. After we won the legislative contest, John called me to congratulate NCPeds for its efforts. His message was, "I had no idea you guys could make all those calls!"

# Child Health Insurance Program (CHIP): The North Carolina Experience

by Dave Tayloe Jr., MD, FAAP; Olson Huff, MD, FAAP; Tom Vitaglione, MPH

In 1995, I was finishing my six years as vice-president/president of NCPeds and still serving as chair of the committee on government affairs (1985–2001). I was completing my sixth year on the AAP Committee on State Government Affairs. During NCPeds' annual meeting, I was asked to meet with the Committee on Children with Special Needs and health insurance administrators whom Committee Chair Adrian Sandler, MD, FAAP, had invited to their meeting. No insurance company administrators showed up. The committee had hoped to convince the insurance plans to provide better coverage for children with special needs who did not qualify for Medicaid.

After this disappointing experience, I called Jim Long, the NC Commissioner of Insurance. (I knew the commissioner and contributed to his re-election campaigns annually.) I asked him to help us set up a meeting with administrators of the major health insurance plans in North Carolina. He appointed a member of his staff, Barbara Morales-Burke, to work with us.

We convened a meeting in the insurance commissioner's office in early 1996 with pediatricians, insurance plan administrators, some state government administrators (including Barbara Matula, the director of Medicaid), and Henry Jones, the lobbyist for NCPeds. After the meeting, the group gave NCPeds direction on drafting legislation that would allow all insurance plans to fairly contribute to a fund to assist special needs children who were ineligible for Medicaid and either uninsured or under-insured.

Our lobbyist drafted the legislation in 1996. The bill called for financial contributions by all health insurance plans that provided insurance for children in NC, based upon the volume of business the plans conducted in the last fiscal year. There would be an official State Commission for Children with Special Needs, made up of representatives of NCPeds and insurance plans. This commission would accept applications for funding and make monetary awards accordingly. The session of the legislature in 1997 would have been the first opportunity to introduce the legislation. However, Congress passed the Balanced Budget Act of 1997, creating the Child Health Insurance Program (CHIP) before we could find legislators to introduce our special needs children bill. We considered our options and decided to wait until we saw what kind of CHIP plan we could develop before pursuing the possibly contentious insurance plan legislation.

The governor appointed a task force to develop a CHIP proposal for the legislature to consider during the next year's legislative session of 1998. I served on the task force with a number of pediatric colleagues and key child advocates. We developed a "Medicaid look-alike" CHIP plan that would be seamless with Medicaid but satisfy federal requirements within the block grant format of CHIP. This proposal was introduced during a special session of the legislature called by Governor Hunt in late March 1998, two months before the regular session of the NC General Assembly was scheduled to begin.

Nothing happened during the first few weeks of this special session, and we discovered that the Republican-controlled House wanted nothing to do with the proposal of the Governor's Task Force. The Republicans wanted CHIP to be a private insurance plan. They were leaning toward putting the CHIP-eligible children into the State Employees' Health Plan, a Blue Cross basic and "bare bones" health insurance plan. We became worried as the days dragged by with no action on CHIP and learned of at least one state that turned down the CHIP opportunity. To us, CHIP was a really big deal!

Before CHIP, the children born into Medicaid whose families' gross annual income were less than or equal to 185 percent of Federal Poverty Guidelines (FPG), would lose Medicaid coverage if their families' gross annual income did not drop to 133 percent or less of FPG by their first birthdays. They lost Medicaid coverage if gross family income did not drop to 100 percent or less of FPG by their sixth birthday. This "stairstep" system (*see illustration*) made it exceedingly difficult for families and physicians to ensure access to care for low-income children. With CHIP, the federal government would give states money to assure that all children born into Medicaid at 200 percent of FPG would remain in Medicaid or CHIP until nineteen years of age. As a block grant program, it would be especially important for states to work with the federal government to assure very accurate estimates of the numbers of CHIP-eligible children. If block grant funding were to run out, the state would have to fund the shortfall or resort to freezing enrollment and/or terminating CHIP-eligible children.

I attended an AAP meeting in Atlanta while the legislature was in session. During that meeting, I talked with a pediatrician friend, Olson Huff, MD, FAAP, NCPeds president at the time, and good friends with a Republican House leader, Representative Lanier Cansler, CPA, from Asheville. Dr. Huff called Representative Cansler and found out that Representative Charlotte Gardner, a retired schoolteacher from Salisbury, was leading the Republican effort on CHIP. I obtained her phone number and, although I did not know her, called her at her home from a pay phone in the meeting hotel lobby. I introduced myself to her as a pediatrician representative of the NCPeds and explained that I understood she was helping lead the effort in the House on CHIP. I explained to her that we were concerned that special needs children might not receive comprehensive services comparable to those covered by Medicaid as administered in the Blue Cross State Employees Plan. She said, "I am so glad you called. We need input from the pediatricians on our bill." She invited Dr. Huff and me to have

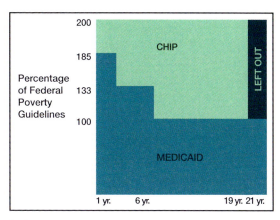

Stairstep system

dinner with her the following Wednesday night in Raleigh. She invited Representative Cansler. We invited Tom Vitaglione, chairperson of the CHIP Task Force and head of Children's Health Services in the Division of Public Health.

During that dinner, the legislators invited us to come to their offices the next day to help amend their bill according to our concerns about services for special needs children. I was on-call in my practice the next day, so Dr. Huff and Mr. Vitaglione took our draft special needs bill and went to the legislative offices the next day. They inserted much of the language from our draft bill on children with special needs into the Republican CHIP bill. The amended bill called for a Commission on Children with Special Needs that would review denied claims to ensure that the CHIP-covered children received benefits comparable to those in Medicaid. Twenty million dollars per year was included as a special fund to pay for services authorized by the Commission.

By the time Dr. Huff and Mr. Vitaglione left the legislators' offices that day, the governor and secretary of Health and Human Services had found out about how the pediatricians were working with the Republican leadership of the House, and they were not happy. Dr. Huff and I had to return to Raleigh the following Monday to "explain ourselves" to the Democratic Senate leadership and governor representatives. Over that weekend, I contacted academic and practicing pediatricians, nineteen in all, to see if they preferred a Medicaid-like CHIP plan or a Blue Cross CHIP plan. Seventeen of the nineteen preferred a Medicaid plan, mainly because they understood Medicaid better than they did private insurance. Because we were afraid that the legislature would go home with no CHIP plan if we "called the bluff" of the Republicans in the House, we decided to tell the Democratic leaders of the Senate and representative of the governor that the NCPeds endorsed the Republican plan. When the senators and governor's representative realized that the pediatricians, who had served on the CHIP Task Force, really were okay with the Blue Cross CHIP plan, they approved the Republican plan, and it passed both the NC House and Senate to become law.

Governor Hunt appointed me to chair the Commission on Children with Special Needs for the first four years of CHIP. This commission reviewed all insurance claims for CHIP children that were denied to make sure the CHIP children received services comparable to those available to Medicaid-eligible children. We were able to amend our CHIP bill during subsequent legislative sessions to the point that we never really needed the special appropriated fund. Our CHIP benefits were very comparable to those of Medicaid. Physicians were happy with our CHIP plan since they were paid private insurance rates, which were significantly higher than Medicaid payments.

To summarize the feelings of NCPeds, President Olson Huff, MD, FAAP, stated:

> Each day in North Carolina, thousands of children who are not eligible for Medicaid and whose families do not earn enough to pay for their own health insurance still have access to the medical care they need because North Carolina's pediatricians made sure that it would happen. When the US Congress passed the Balanced Budget Act in 1997, the Children's Health Insurance Plan, known as CHIP, was established. Thus, the way was paved to close the gap between those eligible for Medicaid and those still not able to pay for health care coverage. Each state was expected to design its own plan to administer funds and enroll eligible recipients, and that was when, in North Carolina, problems erupted.

> A divided NC legislature failed initially to reach an agreement to adopt the new legislation because the House was controlled by a Republican majority, with the Senate dominated by a Democratic majority. Lawmakers were at a stalemate. Lanier Cansler, a member of the House Republicans who asked for pediatricians to help, contacted me. After meeting with him, I contacted Dr. Dave Tayloe Jr. who was in a meeting out of town.

He contacted other members of the House of Representatives from his district, and we subsequently met with a small group of Republicans in Raleigh. Their concern was that CHIP would just become another Medicaid-like program that would add more cost to the state budget.

I met with Democratic leaders in the Senate, but my attempt to bridge the gap met with frustration, and I felt as if they did not think we were supporting the recommendations of the governor's appointed task force to help those who would be eligible for the expanded health coverage. Due to further efforts by Dr. Dave Tayloe Jr. the support of the NCPeds Liaison committee, Tom Vitaglione, and Representative Lanier Cansler in the NC House of Representatives, a plan allowing Medicaid to expand coverage to the population of special needs children and the rest of the eligible pediatric population included in the state health plan was proposed and accepted. There was considerable back and forth in meetings to get this important piece of legislation passed in North Carolina, and the fact that it became a remarkably successful program, now called NC Health Choice, is a direct result of the involvement of North Carolina's pediatricians and their dedication as advocates for the health of the children in our state.

After years of advocacy led by NCPeds and the advocacy organization NC Child, the NC General Assembly agreed to merge NC Health Choice (CHIP) with Medicaid in the 2022 legislative session. Predictably, this action had been one of the original recommendations from NCPeds during the contested political row for NC Health Choice in 1997-98. This long-sought decision was facilitated by the fact that NCPeds had successfully advocated for NC Health Choice benefits almost identical to Medicaid. Thus, when Medicaid Transformation (the transition to a managed-care model) was adopted by the legislature in 2021 as the future direction of Medicaid, there would be no significant cost difference between the programs. This change allowed the managed care plans and NCPeds to convince the General Assembly that it was time to eliminate the confusion of operating two nearly identical programs. After twenty-five years, and following NCPeds' original recommendation of the merger of CHIP into a single Medicaid plan is being implemented effective July 1, 2023.

A harbinger of this change occurred ten years ago in 2012, with the backing of NCPeds, when the Department of Health and Human Services (DHHS) convinced the legislature to shift the administration of NC Health Choice from Blue Cross Blue Shield to the state division of medical assistance. It was demonstrated that by streamlining administration, there were savings for both providers and the state.

Of course, the ultimate beneficiaries are the 100,000-plus children who have gained access to the full Medicaid benefits package and their families who no longer have to deal with the bureaucracy and eccentricities of two programs.

# Part II

## Value of the Executive Director

# Presidents Who Served Before NCPeds Hired an Executive Director, 1978-1998

by Drs. Dave Williams; Bob Schwartz; Steve Edwards; Dave Tayloe Jr.; Olson Huff

## Dave Williams, MD, FAAP, General Pediatrician, Thomasville

I was fortunate to serve as president of NCPeds for the three years that included 1978–1980. I became involved early in my practice in 1969 when Archie Johnson, MD, of the Bowman Gray School of Medicine at Wake Forest University, came to my office and did a "time study." That was my first interaction with Dr. Johnson, and we became good friends. He was elected president of NCPeds in 1975, and I was elected vice president. We traveled to the District IV American Academy of Pediatrics meetings, as I became actively involved with NCPeds at a fairly young age.

When I became president, my first duty was to continue to increase our number of committees as it had been revised by Dr. Johnson. We also worked to increase attendance at our three liaison committee meetings each year. We tried to make sure we had good attendance of practicing pediatricians from across the state, as well as from our academic centers. We enlisted the support of the five chairs of the departments of pediatrics in residency programs at Carolinas Medical Center (Charlotte), Duke University (Durham), East Carolina University (Greenville), University of North Carolina (Chapel Hill), and Wake Forest University (Winston-Salem). In addition, all pediatricians working in different sections of state government were invited, along with non-physician leaders of government children's programs and child advocacy organizations. I felt this was very worthwhile and certainly enhanced our main agenda—to improve the health care and outcomes of children in our state.

Another endeavor brought to completion during my three years as president was the publication of a History of our Pediatric Society, written by Peter English, MD, PhD, an assistant professor of pediatrics and history at Duke University. Also, our friends at UNC and Duke collaborated on producing a child state health plan that was endorsed by Governor Jim Hunt. This proposal's chief premise was that all children should have a medical home in the practice of a pediatrician or family physician.

As far as the day-to-day operation of NCPeds, we did not have a paid executive director, but Mrs. John McClain served as the keeper of our treasury. She kept an index card file of all members and worked out of her home in Durham. Charlie Scott, MD, FAAP, of Burlington, was secretary, and Jim Rouse, MD, FAAP, of Durham, was treasurer. Dr. Rouse and I would meet with Mrs. McClain from time to time in her home to go over membership records and finances. We would try to think of

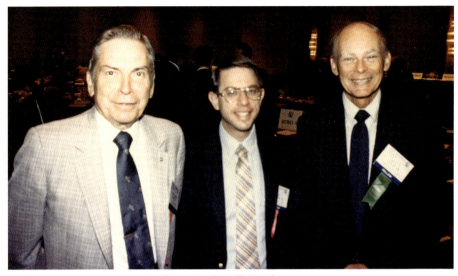

**Left to Right: George Prince, Bob Schwartz, Dave Tayloe Sr.**
**NCPeds Past Presidents, 1986**

pediatricians in the state who were not members, develop a plan to reach out to those pediatricians to invite them to become members, and make sure dues were being paid in a timely manner by all members. This was long before the internet and cell phones were commonplace, so all our work involved face-to-face meetings, telephone calls, and writing and sending "snail-mail" letters and statements. Having no executive director or secretary, I depended upon my office staff to help produce NCPeds' regular bulletins.

### Bob Schwartz, MD, FAAP, Pediatric Endocrinologist at Carolinas Medical Center, Charlotte

I was president of the chapter from 1987–1989 and vice president for George Prince, MD, FAAP, who served as president from 1984–1987. In total, this was a six-year commitment. Planning the annual meeting was a major responsibility. This was done with the support of Carol Russell from the North Carolina Medical Society. I would meet Carol at potential meeting sites, often with my wife, Rebecca, to assess the facilities for size (number of rooms), amenities, opportunities for recreation (golf, tennis, swimming), dining options, and, of course, the cost. Our late-summer annual meetings rotated between the Blockade Runner Hotel in Wrightsville Beach and the Grove Park Inn in Asheville. The pediatric department chairs from Duke University, East Carolina University, the University of North Carolina, and

Wake Forest University rotated the responsibility for choosing the educational topics and speakers for the annual meeting. We also had a spring meeting on the Saturday of the NC Medical Society annual meeting, with an abbreviated education program at The Carolina Hotel in Pinehurst, the famous golf resort. Social events were sponsored by pharmaceutical companies, especially those that made infant formulas. We often had a live band with dancing on Saturday evening. In addition, we had a winter executive committee/liaison committee meeting, usually somewhere mid-state.

We did not have an executive director, but we did have a contract part-time lobbyist and a telephone contact tree where pediatric society members were assigned specific legislators to contact for legislative issues. The contact list was developed in 1983 by executive committee member Frank Gearing, MD, FAAP, and reconfigured by Dave Tayloe Jr., MD, FAAP, chair of the committee on legislation from 1985–2001.

As president, I always attended the AAP National Conference, the annual chapter forum, now the annual leadership forum (ALF), and our district meetings. I tried to be prompt in responding to issues and problems. However, any success in that area was due to the excellent secretaries at Charlotte Memorial Hospital during my term as president.

The most exciting thing that happened during my presidency was the vaccine legislation following the lawsuit involving Dr. David Tayloe Sr. (see *Big Dave: Visionary Leader*) I asked Dave Tayloe Jr., MD, to take over as legislative chair, and he, of course, did an outstanding job, resulting in North Carolina being the first and only state to have a vaccine compensation law. Another result of this accomplishment was that North Carolina received the Large Chapter Award from the American Academy of Pediatrics. Unfortunately, we had a significant deficit due to our expenses related to lobbying for the vaccine legislation. However, we asked for and received twenty-five dollar donations from 85 percent of our chapter members to cover that $10,000 shortfall. In addition, we were able to get one of the pharmaceutical companies producing vaccines to make a significant donation to the chapter.

Having the honor of being the president of NCPeds has been the highlight of my professional career. The friendships I formed with NC pediatricians and other pediatricians in what was then District 4 (NC, SC, TN, KY, VA, GA, FL, PR), as well as the pediatrician leaders and outstanding staff in the American Academy of Pediatrics, have been long-term relationships. It was a good ride!

### Steve Edwards, MD, FAAP, General Pediatrician, Raleigh

I served as chapter president for three years (1990–1992). I had been vice president for three years working with President Robert "Bob" Schwartz, MD. Dave Tayloe Jr., MD, was my vice president. Bob was one of the most organized leaders I had ever met and was, in effect, my mentor for the job. While I had served predecessors in various NCPeds roles for the past twenty years and learned from each of them, Bob was my most important mentor. Bob had nicely described the working situation when I assumed the presidency, so I will not repeat his description.

However, a few things changed slightly. Because I lived in Raleigh, the home of the NC Medical Society office, I was able to meet with Carol Russell, our coordinator from the NC Medical Society, in her office two or three afternoons a month for two or three hours. Carol was excellent at the job for which she was hired. She made all the arrangements for executive committee meetings and our annual educational meetings. She oversaw the quarterly publication of our newsletter, then edited by George Engstrom, MD, FAAP, of Concord, and took tapes of communications from me to individuals and organizations to have them transcribed and mailed to appropriate recipients.

The Blockade Runner in Wilmington was becoming too small for our group and showing a lot of wear and tear. Carol traveled with Bob and me to Morehead City to evaluate several potential new meeting sites. We settled on the Sheraton Hotel at Atlantic Beach as the primary location and contracted with a private club for social events. We continued to meet at the Grove Park Inn on alternate years, but had our annual meeting at the Sheraton for 1990 and 1992.

During the almost weekly meetings with Carol, we discussed future activities for NCPeds. However, Carol primarily saw her role as an implementer of ideas I had garnered from meetings and communications with my executive committee and committee chairs. We communicated regularly with the NC Academy of Family Physicians and met with them several times a year at their office to coordinate common goals. They owned their own building and employed a full-time executive director. The advantages of this arrangement were very obvious, but I struggled with the question of how we could pay for such services. This issue was discussed at executive committee meetings without solutions. We were already struggling financially and had to ask members for supplemental voluntary contributions for recent vaccine legislative successes during Bob's presidency.

I had served as chair of our government services committee since Dr. David Tayloe Sr. had appointed me in 1982. My primary objective had been to improve payment for Medicaid services to enhance access to care for poor children. Payments were so low that pediatricians who saw large numbers of Medicaid patients were being severely punished economically. For a number of years, my committee had met several times a year with representatives of the Department of Human Resources to press for improvement. Each time we met a similar response: "Pediatricians are such nice people. We appreciate what you do, but we just don't have any money." In 1989 Congress passed the Omnibus Budget Reconciliation Act (OBRA-89). It stated, "Payments for Medicaid services should be such that Medicaid patients have

> The friendships made, hard-earned successes obtained, and, most of all, my belief that together, we have developed a health system that leads the nation in delivering excellent health to all our children.

the same access to services as other patients in the same geographic area." I have told his story elsewhere (see *Medicaid Reform: Negotiating with State Government*), but the bottom line is that payment equity became our priority. With the strong support of our executive committee and the help of our lawyers, we were able to negotiate fairer payments.

My activities through NCPeds have been some of the greatest joys of my life because of the friendships made, the hard-earned successes obtained, and, most of all, my belief that together, pediatricians have helped develop a health system that leads the nation in delivering excellent health care to all of our children.

### Dave Tayloe Jr., MD, FAAP, General Pediatrician, Goldsboro

In 1988, Dr. Robert "Bob" Schwartz approached me about running for vice president-elect of NCPeds. He said I was working too hard as chair of the committee on legislation not to get the "perks" that come with being a chapter president/vice president. He explained that the chapter paid for the president, vice president, and their spouses to attend the annual meeting, the other two executive committee/liaison committee meetings, the AAP Annual Meeting (now the NCE), the AAP Spring Meeting, and the District IV meeting. He reinforced his recruitment pitch by adding, "Your wife really deserves the perks," since the meetings all occurred in rather comfortable vacation settings.

Realizing that Bob would not take no for an answer, I took over as vice president in 1989 while still serving as chair of the committee on legislation and as a member of the AAP Committee on State Government Affairs. My three years as president (1993–1995) proved to be the busiest years of my life because I was a full-time pediatrician and call-taker for my expanding independent group practice and a father to four adolescent children. All correspondence was via mail or landline telephone. Carol Russell, our part-time secretary at the NC Medical Society, helped immensely with the organization and logistics of the three meetings a year and keeping the bills paid. Keeping all the councils and committees active and generating reports for the membership was challenging but rewarding.

The major foci of advocacy efforts were Medicaid reorganization under Carolina Access, Medicaid payment of physicians, and immunizations. Pediatricians in leadership worked tirelessly to develop the physician-directed managed care networks of Carolina Access. When the physician-directed networks were pitted against insurance plan health maintenance organizations (HMOs) in Mecklenburg County, the physician-directed networks proved to be far better in the areas of access, quality, and cost-effectiveness. Therefore, Medicaid contracts with the HMOs were terminated in less than two years.

Persistent negotiation with Medicaid administrators to improve physician payment finally produced tangible results. I confided to my dad, Dave Tayloe Sr., MD, FAAP, who had served in the leadership of NCPeds for a number of years and worked diligently and quietly to improve pediatrician payment, "I cannot believe you retired in 1994; that is the first year pediatricians have been paid fairly by the Medicaid program! You deserved to be paid that well during your thirty-nine-year career!"

NCPeds worked closely with Governor Jim Hunt (with the behind-the-scenes assistance of pediatrician Dr. David Bruton, close friend and political ally of the governor), the immunization branch, and the legislature to create the Universal Childhood Vaccine Distribution Program. This program meshed perfectly with the federal Vaccines for Children Program in 1994 to assure all NC children could receive all recommended vaccines in all public and private health care settings and that providers would be paid at the top of the recommended federal immunization

> Pediatricians in leadership worked tirelessly to develop the physician-directed managed care networks of Carolina Access.

administration scale for giving state or federally funded vaccines to all children who did not have adequate insurance coverage for vaccine-related costs. This triumph, which required an annual state appropriation of approximately $8 million, was the result of relentless chapter efforts that began under the leadership of Dr. Bob Schwartz; Dr. Schwartz became president in 1987 in the middle of the vaccine liability crisis when vaccine costs for physicians and patients rose significantly. As chair of the committee on legislation in 1987, he encouraged me to begin working on a free vaccine program for NC that mirrored those in some other states. Our liaison committee meetings and networking really paid off when our immunization branch friends, regular attendees at our liaison committee meetings, figured out how to put the universal program together for our state. Due to these major accomplishments, NCPeds won another Outstanding Chapter Award from the AAP during my tenure as president.[1]

### Olson Huff, MD, FAAP, Developmental Pediatrician, Asheville

I was the last to serve as president of NCPeds without a full-time executive director (1996–1998) and also was the first to transition from a three-year to the present two-year term. My time as president was enormously gifted by the talents and dedication of my predecessors, Drs. Dave Williams, George Prince, Robert "Bob" Schwartz, Steve Edwards, and Dave Tayloe Jr. It was from them that I was able to model my time as president and lean on their legacy that had begun to make NCPeds a major force in the medical care of children and in the state and national policies that shaped that care.

As I reflect then on my time as president, I think of the question that I am often asked, and I am sure many of my colleagues are often asked: Why pediatrics? What made you decide to become a pediatrician?

The answer for me is like watching the expanding circles in a pool of water after one tosses in a rock. Each circle leads to another, connecting the beginning with all that comes afterward. So, it is not just one thing but a series of happenings, hopefully connected, that creates one's response and, therefore, the ultimate

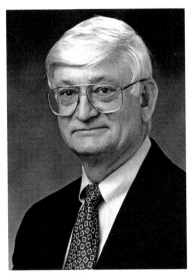

Olson Huff, MD, FAAP

result. That is how I viewed my time as president. My task and my opportunity were to track those circles and to do so as efficiently as possible. As I am more visionary than organized, I had to depend heavily on others to help me.

Dave Rock, former Ross-Abbott Laboratories representative and the first executive director of NCPeds, came along at the end of my term and was of tremendous help in attending to details, helping with the meetings, coordinating agendas, and keeping pace with legislative events. As I was probably the first president to be farther from Raleigh—and since cell phones, texting, and the internet were just emerging—having connections with other parts of the state were vital. I especially relied on the

---

[1] A chapter was ineligible to receive the Outstanding Chapter Award for the three years after it won the award, explaining the AAP principle that one chapter should not dominate as the winner of the prestigious award.

committees and made every effort to communicate with the chairs of each committee and give them time to meet and report at the annual meeting. The Good for Kids Award was initiated to recognize individual advocacy. Among the first recipients were Paula Wolf, child advocate and lobbyist, and Dr. Adrian Sandler, who secured funds for gunlocks that were distributed in Buncombe County.

I was pleased to have the opportunity to work with Dr. Jane Foy. As vice president, she acted as liaison to the pediatric department chairs, helped me establish meeting agendas, and encouraged committee activity and support. Her administrative skills were a major advantage for NCPeds!

Like concentric circles, many issues presented as markers of changes in preventive health and medical care for children. These included, but in no way were limited to, dental care for children, obesity and nutrition, child safety restraints, teen smoking prevention campaigns, mental health parity, child abuse prevention, Medicaid reimbursement, and, of course, the passage of the Child Health Insurance Program legislation. My task in all of this was to coordinate individual and committee actions and to try to keep track of as much of it as possible. Dealing with increasing policy issues that required legislative action began to occupy more of my time and thought.

Establishing the agendas for the executive committee and annual meetings largely on my own was a challenge. I spent many hours before each of those meetings to ensure as much proficiency as possible.

When Dave Rock came on board, many details of daily operations shifted to him, and I was freer to think about the future possibilities and sense where all those circles were moving and merging. I remember when I became president, Dr. Williams told me it would be one of the best experiences imaginable and the friends I would make and colleagues I encountered would greatly enrich my life. He was indeed correct!

# Presidents Who Served After NCPeds Hired an Executive Director

by Drs. Jane Meschan Foy; Bill Hubbard; Chuck Willson; Peter Morris; Herb Clegg; Marian Earls; Karen Breach; John Rusher; Debbie Ainsworth; Scott St. Clair; Susan Mims; Christoph Diasio

## Jane Meschan Foy, MD, FAAP, General Pediatrician, Greensboro and Winston-Salem

My vantage point as chapter president from 1998-2000 was unique in several ways: I was the first chapter president to have a two-year term instead of three-year, the only one to have three executives, and the first (as far as I know) to operate on a deficit budget, using carryover funds to finance the new executive directors. (The latter was

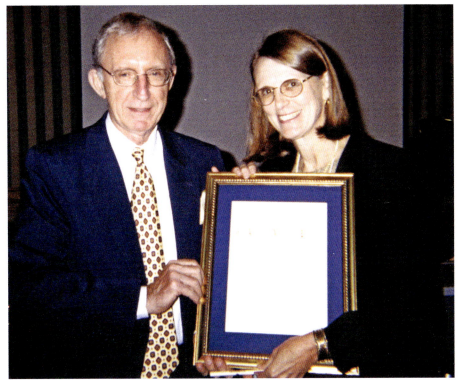

**Richard Perruzi, Director of NC Medicaid, receives recognition from NC Peds President Jane Meschan Foy, MD, FAAP**

an unfortunate coincidence with my also being the first woman president of NCPeds in forty years.) I began with Carol Russell of the NC Medical Society as staff, then had Dave Rock for one year as executive director, then hired and onboarded Steve Shore. Despite the chaos, we were able to form our practice managers' group and education committee; establish our NCPeds Foundation (a non-profit that would help us to generate non-dues revenue); participate in implementation of a Robert Wood Johnson Foundation grant to facilitate outreach and enrollment for the new NC Health Choice insurance program; establish a physicians' advisory group to shepherd Health Choice; form a task force that resulted in dramatically changing NC Medicaid policy and payment for the mental health services provided to children in primary care and school settings; and win an AAP Outstanding Large Chapter Award in the process. My NCPeds workload was huge during that period, but I received tremendous support from Bill Hubbard, vice president/president-elect, and both of us were energized by having our own executive director. Steve helped us eliminate our budget deficit by the end of his first year!

We should give credit to Dave Rock, who organized and energized our practice managers during his year with us; then Steve worked with Bill to take the practice managers' group to the next level. I have always felt that the high level of involvement of practice managers in NCPeds has ensured that our advocacy was grounded in pragmatism and that new policies and programs could be readily translated into practice. NC Health Choice implementation was a prime example.

I agree with everybody's comments that hiring Steve as executive director, and then Elizabeth Hudgins to follow Steve, greatly enhanced our potential to impact state government affairs. I would add that they did not simply take over as lobbyists for NCPeds (which they could well have done, because they came to us with great relationships and talents): they made a point of fostering our members' and leaders' relationships with lawmakers and state government leaders. This has always been NCPeds' special advocacy sauce!

### Bill Hubbard, MD, FAAP, General Pediatrician, Raleigh

I served a two-year term as NCPeds vice president (VP) in 1999 and 2000. Jane Foy was president. She included me in all aspects of chapter business. She was a great mentor for my following two years as president. We had an easy working relationship and became great friends.

My largest responsibility as VP was planning the annual meeting. Carol Russell had retired from the NC Medical Society, Dave Rock resigned, and there was a gap before Steve Shore was hired. The staff assigned to us after Carol retired were Alan Skipper and Patrick Kennedy. They helped me plan our annual meeting in Myrtle Beach. That situation worked okay but was certainly not optimal. I think that period convinced us that NCPeds needed a full-time executive director.

Jane and I served as a search committee. Steve Shore came highly recommended by several NCPeds friends in state government. We met Steve at the NC Academy of Family Physicians headquarters in Raleigh, and we were convinced he was the right choice, which he clearly proved to be!

Assuming the presidency was intimidating, especially considering the leaders who preceded me. They were a hard act to follow. Nevertheless, my leadership years proved to be a rich and meaningful time in my life.

I recall several initiatives during my presidency. There was concern that relatively few academic pediatricians were active chapter members. Several of the academic centers even paid the annual chapter dues for their entire faculty. Nevertheless, there was minimal chapter involvement. In an attempt to convince academic pediatricians that we were doing important work for the welfare of children and that their participation would be valuable, I arranged, through the pediatric department chairs, to do grand rounds to make our case at each institution. Steve Shore made my slides and together we traveled to all the academic medical centers. Steve and I solidified our friendship bond by finding the best barbecue place in each city after the programs.

Wally Brown deserves credit for another initiative during my presidency. The state legislature was trying to determine how they would choose to participate in the CHIP program. I asked Wally to work with Tom Vitaglione to establish a task force made up of providers and representatives of state agencies involved in child welfare to develop a plan to recommend to the legislature. Wally recalls insisting on a round table.

The task force worked great and ultimately recommended the legislature have the CHIP program offer the same benefits to children that are offered in the state employee health insurance plan. This included comparable reimbursement to providers. The end product, named NC Health Choice, we judged to be the best CHIP program in the country. Through Wally, the NCPeds' advocacy made a significant difference.

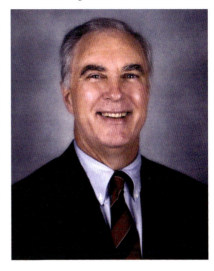

**Dave Rock**

I always remembered Steve Edwards' statement that the well-being of children is dependent on the well-being of their caretakers, which includes their doctors, plus the ability of the families to assure the children have access to the doctors. Annually, pediatricians wrangled with insurance companies over fair reimbursement for services and procedures provided. Communication between providers and payers was frustrating, and results were inconsistent. To improve this interface, I formed the managed care solutions committee. I arranged to get the chair of the pediatric division of each of the major managed care companies to meet monthly with a group of pediatricians to discuss reimbursement and encounter form denial issues. For several years these face-to-face meetings succeeded in improving understanding and mutually beneficial agreements.

### Chuck Willson, MD, FAAP, General Pediatrician, Greenville (private practice for eighteen years followed by many years on faculty at the Brody School of Medicine at East Carolina University)

Child advocacy is a full-time job. Events that affect the lives of children positively and negatively are happening all the time, to say nothing of long struggles with the NC legislature to protect Medicaid coverage and health services for children. By coming together in the NC Pediatric Society, pediatricians joined hands to get the job done.

Child advocacy needs to be someone's full-time job. Our capacity to advocate for kids effectively was greatly enhanced when we rented an office and hired a full-time executive director. During my term as president of NCPeds, I was blessed to work with Steve Shore as our executive director. With a degree in social sciences from Duke University, Steve was well prepared for the job. But it was his heart and compassion that made him outstanding. He really embraced our advocacy mission. He worked tirelessly to be sure that our voices were heard on important issues at the legislature. He hired superb staff with our limited resources and would rather have a new part-time staff member than a raise in his salary. Steve managed our annual meetings and open forums. During his time as executive director, our society won the AAP Very Large Outstanding Chapter Award on two occasions. During my tenure as president, North Carolina was recognized as having the best immunization rates for five-year-old children. I met Governor Easley's wife in Raleigh at a McDonald's to receive the award.

Serving as president of the NCPeds was a great honor, but any success I had was built upon the magnificent work of the pediatricians who served before me. They are my heroes. One of my proudest moments was receiving the AAP Outstanding Large Chapter Award on behalf of NCPeds. I sincerely thank Steve Shore for keeping me on track and strengthening our advocacy for children!

**Peter J. Morris, MD, MPH, MDiv, FAAP, FACPM, Pediatrics, One-Time Pediatric Hospitalist, Public Health Medical Director, Preventive Medicine, Executive Director of Urban Ministries of Wake County**

I do not feel as if I was the first choice to be president-elect my year, as it was a busy time for the best and the brightest of the society. I remember telling Bill Hubbard and Chuck Willson that if no one else had the time to stand for election I thought I could do it. Both Bill and Chuck were individuals who I trusted and with whom I had solid relationships. They had mentored me back to my medical student and residency days.

I have been asked many times in my leadership positions which was more important—knowledge, skills, or relationships—and without hesitation, I always answer relationships!

As I began my apprenticeship as president-elect, Bill and Chuck challenged me to wonder how to recruit younger members, women, and black and brown members. They made me wonder what our pitch to a newer generation of pediatricians was— pediatricians who valued family and private time but still were driven to change the world for their children and the children and families they cared for day in and day out. I listened, watched, and learned, and though it was more than a little corny, it seemed that we pediatricians were full of heart, and if we had a fault, it was we felt so deeply about the injustice and inequity we witnessed each day that we hurt.

I coined the acronym FEALL as my pitch. NCPeds offers fellowship beyond the walls of our insular practices; education within our state with friends we knew from our residencies and friends we ought to know from across town or the next town or the medical center where we knew names but not faces; a place to lift our voices in advocacy because public policy can lift our voices together to save lives and provide leadership in and beyond our communities; leaving a legacy for our children and our children's children. I reached out. I made phone calls. I suggested we could meet by phone or email and still have time for our families. I invited people to as large a role as they were willing to take, perhaps sooner than some of them realized what it might mean. Of course, they rose to the occasion, whatever it was, because passion and experience are the basics of storytelling. And we have stories to tell. Stories that move people to action.

Living in Raleigh, I knew I might be called on before, during, and after my presidency to represent NCPeds in all sorts of forums. I served on the NC Child Fatality Task Force, co-chairing it for a time, and other ad hoc committees, answering legislative questions of the moment. But really, I was building relationships.

No one helped in this quite as much as Steve Shore and Elizabeth Hudgins. Think what you might about what an executive director does—and I am an executive director of a nonprofit these days—but for all the organizing, or meeting work you think we might do, we are really in the business of putting people together in a room to get something done. We are in the relationship business, matching storytellers with people who need to hear stories. Steve and Elizabeth would call and ask if I could be somewhere, and, if I could, I liked it best if they could pick me up from my office so we could talk on the way. That way I could listen, learn, get there early, watch and see, and when it was my turn to share, tell a story making the points I'd been prepared to make. Steve and Elizabeth knew the issue, the players, and the points to make. My task was to make them come alive the way a pediatrician might, with a story that might touch a heart string, a fact that would be shocking but true, and a remedy that was within reach.

So, I think NCPeds is about how we feel, or perhaps FEALL, but certainly about how we come to be in relationship with one another, with the children and families we serve, and with the future we are trying to shape and create with the help of others.

## Herb Clegg, MD, FAAP, General Pediatrician/Pediatric Infectious Diseases, Charlotte

Having a full-time executive director, and, in particular, Steve Shore, gave NCPeds much greater access to the state legislature, the NC Medical Society, and the NC Academy of Family Physicians because of Steve's long-standing connections with influential groups, individuals within state government, and public health leaders.

He connected in a much more engaging way with our academic partners, and drew in academic pediatricians, not just department chairpersons. His organizational ability empowered him to strengthen the practice managers' section.

He certainly helped me stay organized, and arranged for me to travel to different academic centers to discuss NCPeds and to juggle a number of different programs NCPeds had going on during my term as president.

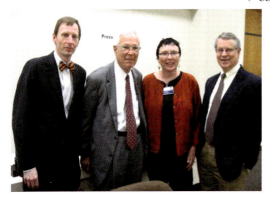

Left to Right: Henry Jones Jr., JD; William R. Purcell, MD, FAAP; Marian Earls, MD, MTS, FAAP; Herb Clegg, MD, FAAP

### Marian Earls, MD, MTS, FAAP, Developmental Pediatrician, Greensboro

My leadership roles for the NC Pediatric Society spanned a number of years—as secretary, chair of the mental health committee, vice president, and president (2008–2010). For years then, I had the great benefit of the NCPeds legacy of relationship building with state organizations and government, and I had the responsibility of maintaining that legacy. For all of those years, Steve Shore was the executive director. Steve had excellent skills in building relationships and facilitating them for NC Pediatric Society leaders.

In 2001, while working on children's mental health, we were able to achieve a Medicaid policy that, for children receiving mental health services, the first six visits can have a non-specific diagnosis code. This recognizes that for children with emerging symptoms, establishing a diagnosis requires several visits for assessment. It also recognizes that some children have functional concerns that will not rise to the level of the Diagnostic and Statistical Manual of Mental Disorders (DSM-5).

In 2008, Steve Shore worked with me on a white paper about children and adolescents in foster care and their need for follow-up of social-emotional development, continuity, and a medical home. His support and vetting of that white paper resulted in funding from The Duke Endowment and collaboration with the Department of Social Services (DSS), Medicaid, community organizations, mental health professionals, and Community Care of NC (CCNC).

This collaboration has led to policy development to achieve standards of care through the Fostering Health NC program. Steve's successor, Elizabeth Hudgins, helped work to then establish the contract between DSS and NCPeds for the Fostering Health NC work.

For the president of the society to be in practice, or to be faculty, outside of Raleigh is the situation most of the time for the NCPeds. The executive director assures the presence of NCPeds for policy and legislative advocacy, even when the president cannot be present. The executive director also provides continuity as leadership transitions every two years. Most importantly, we have had the good fortune of executive directors with excellent skill sets, and executive directors who are true partners in developing and implementing the evolving agenda of NCPeds.

## Karen Breach, MD, FAAP, General Pediatrician, Charlotte

I was honored to serve as president of the North Carolina chapter of the AAP from 2010–2012. I began my tenure on the board of directors in 2004, ascending the ranks under the leadership of Presidents Peter Morris, Herb Clegg, Marian Earls, and,

of course, our longtime executive director, Steve Shore. The chapter was a well-oiled machine, and I should have felt no pressure upon my election. Having been a recent recipient of the AAPs highest chapter honor, we were not eligible for another AAP award during my term of office. Although Steve was contemplating retirement, he was there for my administration. No pressure.

Well, there was pressure—the greatest of which was to "never let them see me sweat" in my obvious, unspoken position. I was the first African American president of NCPeds. As my good friend and

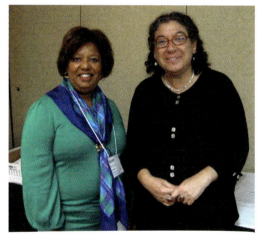

Dr. Karen Breach, NCPed's first African American President with Dr. Perri Klass, National Medical Director of Reach Out and Read, at the 2012 Annual Meeting, Wilmington, NC.

mentor, Dr. Renee Jenkins (past AAP president) said after she was elected: "This is a really big deal." I silently beamed with pride as I saw minority physician membership and overall meeting attendance grow during these years.

Our chapter program was strong as we offered more CME each year. We focused on programs supported by the NCPeds Foundation: foster care, and Healthy and Ready to Learn. We grew the charitable giving from the chapter membership, implemented grant funding, and began to explore the possibility of combining our chapter and foundation operations under a single tax entity to do more for the children of North Carolina.

A focus on chapter operations was a priority for my administration. We moved into a more electronic world, and the last of the handwritten membership rosters, which were most meticulously managed by Dr. Dave Williams, were entered into the electronic database. We adopted new chapter bylaws. Because things did not have to be done the way they always had, committees and meetings were restructured and reorganized. The goal was to streamline meetings to conduct the business of the chapter more efficiently. An added benefit of a more efficient meeting was the opportunity for more social and networking time for the board members and past presidents after the business meeting.

During my administration, I traversed almost the entire state for open forums and meetings. Not being a North Carolina native, I enjoyed my field trips around the state, meeting and engaging more of our members, and learning more about our 100 counties.

My year as immediate past president was also very impactful. Steve Shore really did announce his retirement, and I had the responsibility of chairing the search committee for his replacement. I am proud to say that we selected Elizabeth Hudgins who has not missed a beat since becoming our executive director.

My position in the chapter opened other doors of opportunities to serve in the AAP. Following my presidency, I was honored to be elected to serve as the District IV representative to the national nominating committee for three years.

While we did not win any AAP chapter awards, we put the work in for the children, families, and child health professionals of North Carolina. I would also like to believe I left a positive impact on my younger colleagues as a role model. In the words of my sorority sister, vice president of the United States, Kamala Harris, "I may be the first, but I certainly won't be the last."

It has been my honor to serve as a leader of NCPeds, the North Carolina Chapter of the American Academy of Pediatrics.

### John Rusher, MD, FAAP, General Pediatrician, Raleigh

I served as the president of NCPeds, over a two-year term from 2012 to 2014. I had the pleasure of working with two full-time executive directors: Steve Shore, who retired at the end of my term after fifteen years of service, and Elizabeth Hudgins, who was hired in 2014 and serves as our current executive director.

I cannot understate the outstanding value and reputation that these executive directors have generated for NCPeds during their tenures. Our society has grown in membership and influence as we worked to improve the lives of all children, and the lives of the pediatric providers who care for them. Our executive directors, and the staff that works with them, have guided us to becoming a mature and effective nonprofit organization.

I cannot understate the outstanding value and reputation that these executive directors have generated for NCPeds during their tenures.

**Financial Stability:** With the help of Kim Day, our part-time certified public accountant (CPA), we formalized the status of the NCPeds Foundation as the charitable arm of the society. That nonprofit, whose assets are now managed by the NC Community Foundation, has enabled NCPeds to attract grants and charitable contributions. This, in turn, expands our revenue opportunities and makes the society less reliant on membership dues as our only source of income.

**Stability of Infrastructure:** After several strategic planning sessions led by the executive committee, the officers, and our executive director, we continued to strengthen the committee structure for NCPeds. That structure ensures continuity of the key programs of NCPeds, including the open forum meetings, efforts to prioritize policy issues, and outreach activities across the state.

**Expanded Advocacy:** During my term, our advocacy efforts were forced to shift from the General Assembly to the NC Division of Medical Assistance (DMA) (Medicaid) when the delay in provider payments—secondary to problems with conversion to NC Tracks, the new payment computer payment system—put many pediatric practices across the state into financial crises that threatened their ongoing viability. We were able to secure some emergency funds from NC Department of Health and Human Services (DHHS) for these practices as the payment system recovered. As a result, NCPeds continues to meet, often monthly, with DMA administrators to address issues around child health care, fiscal responsibility, and practice solutions for pediatric providers, issues that have become particularly important during recent times of Medicaid transformation. The full-time executive director is the critical source of continuity in these discussions, working both with the NCPeds board members and with our collaborative partners such as the NC Academy of Family Physicians and the NC Psychiatric Association.

As I look at the many successes of NCPeds over the years, it is clear to me that while many pediatricians have made significant contributions to the organization and the children, families, and pediatricians it serves, none of it could have happened without the glue that comes from our strong executive directors and their dedicated staff.

## Debbie Ainsworth, MD, FAAP, General Pediatrician, Washington

I remember sitting with John Rusher on a bus heading from Arlington, Virginia, to Washington, DC, for a district AAP meeting. I was starting my second year as vice president, and he was finishing his second year of being president. He told me that Steve Shore, our only executive director, would be retiring within the year. I was crushed. All that I had counted on for support as a newbie president just went down the drain.

Karen Breach-Washington, the most recent past president, was the chair of the search committee for a new executive director. The committee honored me by inviting me to participate in the final interview process for selecting an executive director. The decision from that committee was to hire Elizabeth Hudgins. Her passion and her lobbying experience from previous jobs made her perfect for our executive director role. So, she and I started off together in the fall of 2014, leading NCPeds. We got blasted with the usual legislative stuff, but also Medicaid transformation and the "Bathroom Bill," House Bill 2. Elizabeth's skills and connections with legislators were key to our inroads to making changes to various legislative proposals. While we were not successful in defeating the Medicaid reform bill, her leadership, for years, has kept pediatricians in the forefront, making us better prepared for whatever issues may arise next. The following years have accentuated her importance to the success of the NCPeds. Most recently with the COVID-19 issues, her immediate response to start "Solutions Share," an open Zoom meeting every Tuesday at 5:30 p.m., has pulled us all together and given us a forum in which to share current experiences and obtain information about impending crises. Plus, during these stressful times, we benefit from sharing our troubles with like-minded professionals during these very uplifting sessions.

## Scott St. Clair, MD, FAAP, General Pediatrician, Boone

I was blessed during my tenure to have Elizabeth Hudgins as our executive director. In summary, we could not have done any of the society's work during my time as president without her.

As I came in as president, we were dealing with two critical issues. First, we faced down the issue of vaccine administration reimbursement. Briefly, DMA was contractually obligated to pay a certain amount for vaccine administration during the "bump years" of the Affordable Care Act, but ended up paying less. This amounted to a significant decrease in revenue to practices for a critical public health service. The society had to make the difficult choice to file a lawsuit against DMA, while at the same time maintaining our long-standing working relationship with them. We won the lawsuit and continued our good relationship with DMA; this was only possible because of the behind the scenes work by Elizabeth.

The second major issue was Medicaid transformation. While we were not happy about private insurance plans taking over Medicaid, we spent considerable time working with officials within Medicaid to connect with our pediatric council and members about making this transition happen as smoothly as possible for practitioners and patients. Elizabeth made this all work.

In addition, we had things come our way (as they inevitably do!) during my time as president. Two things stand out. The Trump administration and Congress proposed a block grant for Medicaid that would have had a significant negative impact on millions of Medicaid recipients. With Elizabeth's help, we organized a substantial effort to call our North Carolina legislators to block this action. This was eventually defeated with the decisive vote of John McCain. The other major event was Hurricane Florence, which forced us to cancel our annual meeting (this was before COVID-19 and the first time the society had canceled this event). Elizabeth helped steer us through that, and, due to outstanding planning and follow through, was able to use insurance to obtain a refund of the money we had paid up front when planning the event.

I am grateful for my time as president, but it would not have been at all possible without the outstanding work of our executive director!

### Susan Mims, MD, MPH, FAAP, General Pediatrician, Asheville

My presidency began in a hurricane when we had to cancel the annual meeting for the first time in NCPeds history due to the storm on the coast. We still made money on the event because our brilliant staff thought to purchase insurance with a force majeure clause! My presidency ended in the COVID-19 pandemic with our first-ever virtual annual meeting! Fortunately, there were some less turbulent times in the middle, but not many as the society prepared for Medicaid transformation, filed lawsuits against the state, expanded membership and development, and advocated (as our long history has trained us to do) for policies supporting kids and the providers who care for them.

While assuming the role of NCPeds president was a daunting task, it was made easier because of a well-established system of mentorship. Mine came from so many before me including: Dr. Olson Huff, the reason I became involved in NCPeds and a tireless advocate for children; Dr. Peter Morris, who was always ready with questions to get me headed in the right direction; Dr. Marian Earls, who always has something to help my cough; Dr. John Rusher, an intellectual thought-partner; Dr. Debbie Ainsworth, who brought endless passion to the effort; and Dr. Scott St. Clair, who helped me learn the ropes as I served as vice president during his tenure as president.

Despite the challenging beginning and end to my time in the president's office, we accomplished a great deal through the contributions of so many dedicated members and an amazing staff. None of this would have been possible without Elizabeth Hudgins, our executive director. Her dedication and commitment are as never-ending as the ideas of our pediatrician members for ways to improve the health of children. Fortunately, Elizabeth brings much needed realism, practicality, and organizational skills to ensure the society takes on what we can accomplish so we deliver on what we commit to do. She not only goes above and beyond in her role, but she also orchestrates and supports an incredible team. During my presidency year, we took a leap of faith to hire a staff member to focus on our development and membership efforts. Expanding membership, grant writing, and giving options for donating money to NCPeds through an annual campaign and planned-giving (with the help of Dr. Rusher) paid off with increased membership dues and philanthropic support. This increase more than covered the cost of the new position and allowed the society to take advantage of important advocacy opportunities when they presented and to do even more to help North Carolina's children.

> NCPeds could not have supported the pediatricians across our state (members or not) without our dedicated staff team.

With Elizabeth's help and our growing staff, we were able to add committees and task forces to address important issues such as engaging subspecialists in membership and leadership and incorporating an intentional focus on equity, diversity, and inclusion, not only in membership and board composition, but also in all aspects of NCPeds work (education, programs, and advocacy). I had the pleasure of representing NCPeds to receive the AAP Outstanding Very Large Chapter Award in 2020. Our executive director and our staff are the ones who harness the work of as many members as possible to get this type of recognition and, more importantly, to successfully promote better outcomes for our children!

My second year was consumed with responding to the COVID-19 pandemic and helping pediatricians survive it. It is hard to explain all that our staff, led by Elizabeth, orchestrated to ensure pediatricians had accurate information, a means to have their voices heard, financial support to continue to offer care, protective equipment, educational materials, support for virtual care, and most importantly, emotional sustenance through this incredibly trying time. NCPeds could not have supported the pediatricians across our state (members or not) without our dedicated staff team.

This was an "all in" time and I know the children in our state received better care because of their efforts. I get a bit emotional even writing this, and simply cannot thank them enough!

### Christoph Diasio, MD, FAAP, General Pediatrician, Southern Pines

The executive director and professional staff enable the amazing work of NCPeds. My involvement with NCPeds began as pediatric council co-chair when Steve Shore was the executive director, so I have not ever known NCPeds without an executive director. I was immediately impressed by how the executive director can convert multiple wishes of pediatricians, like "wouldn't it be good for children if we could only..." into successful advocacy efforts.

I was eager to be president in the transformation of Medicaid Direct into private insurance company (Prepaid Health Plan (PHP) Medicaid because NCPeds needed to be proactive to limit the negative consequences for children, families, and pediatricians—but I did not realize we would also have to fight a global COVID-19 pandemic at the same time!

These immense challenges have brought out the best in NCPeds, and I have been continuously impressed by the connections our executive director Elizabeth Hudgins is able to make so we can advocate for children's health with key decision-makers in state government. Elizabeth had the terrific idea to create a weekly "Solution Share" during COVID-19 so that members could gather on Zoom once a week at 5:30 PM on Tuesdays to share best practices and good ideas. This has served as a ready-made focus group when state leaders have had ideas to share with NCPeds or needed pediatricians' advice on important policy decisions. One of our solution shares identified an unanticipated problem with Medicaid transformation in July 2021 when the hospitals canceled pre-scheduled operating room cases for dental restorations because the PHPs were requiring prior authorizations (PAs) before they would pay for the procedures. This PA process was not required under traditional Medicaid, so pediatric dentists had to reschedule patients while they figured out how to navigate the cumbersome PA process. After the solution share discussion, Elizabeth and NCPeds were able to rapidly solve this problem through collaboration with DHHS Medicaid administrators and all the PHPs.

As president of the society, I conducted a standing weekly hour-long call with Elizabeth, during which we planned the week ahead, prioritized urgent problems, and developed possible strategies. I developed a heartfelt appreciation for the work of the entire NCPeds staff. It is remarkable how much our staff does on behalf of children on a small budget! It is critical that NCPeds leaders and members realize just how much is being done by the staff. The main reason our leaders often look good and in command of the issues is the amazing relationships our staff has built with partners in government and the child advocacy community as well as the virtual and face-to-face meetings the staff attends on our behalf.

*Editor's Note: I do not think many of us understood how lucky we were to have developed our NCPeds infrastructure until we confronted the COVID-19 pandemic and Medicaid transformation simultaneously. Our current president, our executive director, and our staff have utilized this infrastructure to assure NCPeds could take its members to the next level, and successfully navigate our way through these two unprecedented crises. We should be forever grateful for the amazing work of President Christoph Diasio and executive director Elizabeth Hudgins, and for the efforts of all previous leaders for developing the remarkably effective infrastructure of NCPeds.*

## Steward of Advocacy: The Chapter Executive

by Steve Shore, MSW

**NCPEDS EXECUTIVE DIRECTOR 1999-2014**

There was a "transition moment" during my September 1999 job interview with NCPeds when I knew that I had a very good chance of being recommended for the position of executive director. The chapter received assistance for meeting planning and some administrative help from the NC Medical Society beginning in the 1980s. As the chapter gained members in the early 1990s, discussion started about having a dedicated staff to manage the organization's affairs. Leadership tested the waters with a contractual executive arrangement for one year beginning in 1998. Dave Rock, a retired Abbott Labs employee, handled the duties, and, just one year later, Rock's experience helped determine that the time had come to take the next step and officially hire a full-time executive director.

As President Jane Foy and Vice President Bill Hubbard conducted the interview, our mutual interests began to converge on the vital mission to improve health care access and outcomes tempered by a healthy respect for boosting the business model that allows members to be successful in practice and to be strong voices for children. My practice management experience was an asset, along with my federal and state lobbying work on behalf of community and migrant health centers. This unmistakable expression of advocacy as a primary mission of NCPeds became the dominant topic of the interview and was the major selling point for me. I departed the interview with a vision of managing the organizational resources in a manner that would extend the advocacy outreach of pediatricians, individually and collectively. Another asset in place was the fledgling practice managers network started by Rock, which turned into a powerhouse of practical assistance and collaboration when

NCPeds launched the first two-way listserv communications tool for managers. The match—the NCPed's mission and my experience—was affirmed by the executive committee at the September 1999 annual meeting, and I began my fifteen-year tenure, retiring at the close of 2014.

The executive director of any professional association, and especially those organized by physicians, will wear many hats in the roles of planning and directing meetings, creating publications and programs that favor the priorities of the leadership and members, plus representing pediatricians in numerous public and private settings before large and small groups. There is also the accountability for managing overall operations, especially fiscal resources, ethically and in compliance with state and federal laws and regulations. A desirable trait is the ability to connect and negotiate with advocacy organizations who find common cause with pediatricians to improve child and adolescent health care and outcomes. The chapter became a significant player in multiple collaborative ventures with the full blessing of the leadership and members. This is why it is easy to say that no role was more gratifying during my tenure as executive director than wearing the advocacy hat.

> Valuable alliances were cultivated among our usual, and sometimes unusual, allies.

Pediatricians are prevention minded by intentional training and are encouraged to take an active professional leadership role from the top down. Both the American Academy of Pediatrics (the North American professional membership organization for pediatricians) and the American Board of Pediatrics (the credentialing organization that certifies a high level of physician competence) strongly promote advocacy coaching and experience during a pediatrician's educational journey. Medical students, residents, and fellows are always invited to participate in our advocacy affairs. I relished the challenge of directing the energy and effort to focus our fiscal and human resources to accomplish chapter goals and objectives and the commitment and energy of our members. Valuable alliances were cultivated among our usual, and sometimes unusual, allies. On many occasions, the stakes were high and the outcomes unpredictable, especially when legislative or regulatory change was on the table with the administrative or legislative branches of government. Through it all, NCPeds used its brand, diverse child health expertise,

On many occasions, the stakes were high and the outcomes unpredictable, especially when legislative or regulatory change was on the table with the administrative or legislative branches of government.

geographic dispersion, and the unselfish willingness of members to take on a variety of advocacy challenges.

The founding of the American Academy of Pediatrics in 1930 was an intentional act of advocacy for pediatricians and for children, the consequences of which have conclusively influenced family life, clinical medicine, and health care, not only for the United States but the global community. Times were simpler in the 1930s with just over half of all Americans living in small cities or rural areas and twenty percent of the labor force engaged in farming. The twentieth century started with a profound transformation in the training of physicians by requiring all medical schools to convert from two-year to four-year curricula. This also helped usher in the formalization of specialties in medicine. It has been demonstrated that knowledge, technology, and application began to double every ten years after the Second World War. In 2021, the doubling of knowledge is now said to occur every eighteen months and for technology, every fifteen months. Hardware and software were once exotic terms that are now established in the lexicon of medical practice.

So much has changed in America over the ninety years since the Academy was founded, but the physical, emotional, and psychosocial needs of children and families and the pediatricians who serve them are remarkably similar. An examination of almost any American textbook of pediatrics from the eighteenth to the twenty-first centuries will reveal this comparability. Perhaps no one realized in 1930 how pediatricians would respond and move forward to gain recognition as one of America's foremost child advocacy organizations. The Academy and state chapters have sought to institutionalize responsive modernization and improvement in medical treatment, preventive health care and clinical research, home life, school, the natural environment, and wherever children, adolescents, and their families experience life. NCPeds embraced this movement and demonstrated many times over the persuasive capacity of pediatricians as advocates.

# Advocacy Reflections: Executive Director

**by Elizabeth Hudgins, MPP**

**NCPEDS EXECUTIVE DIRECTOR 2014-PRESENT**

I was honored to join NCPeds as executive director in 2014. As an NC native working in the state's child and family policy advocacy space for the previous decade, I was well acquainted with the strong work of NCPeds and the terrific leadership of Steve Shore, MSW. I quickly realized just how wonderful the full membership is and the tremendous history and passion pediatricians bring to advocacy.

NC is special with its sustained and strategic focus on policies to improve the lives of children and families: In previous jobs, I headed the state Kids Count project in both Arizona (where my husband's first job took us in the late 1990s) and North Carolina (once we were able to return home in 2005).

In examining the state rankings, I realized that a state might tick up or down a few notches, but basically, states at the bottom stayed at the bottom, states in the middle stayed in the middle, etc. One rare exception was a substantial gain North Carolina achieved in reducing child deaths (ages one to seventeen). While in Arizona, I called some folks in North Carolina, but nobody could tell me why. Once I got back, I realized why: There was no single-dose answer but rather a sustained and strategic focus on the issue. Road safety laws helped, but that was just a piece. Careful attention to child nutrition programs helped, but also just a piece. Immediate and strong implementation of the Child Health Insurance Program (CHIP) helped, but it, too, was just a piece. Widespread acceptance by pediatricians of Medicaid helped a lot, but it was still a piece of the puzzle. All of these policies—and more—working together is what created that profound difference. Critically, it was also all these people working together that made a difference.

The top advocacy award for NCPeds is named for "civilian" Tom Vitaglione, who worked at the division of public health and NC Child. NC Child has always had a pediatrician on its board, and pediatric luminaries such as Doctors Olson Huff and Dave Tayloe Jr. have served as senior fellows. The NC Division of Public Health has pediatricians serving in key leadership positions. Working together to keep a sustained and strategic focus on child health has made an important difference for families in NC.

The elements of successful advocacy have changed and are changing more, but relationships are forever. My 1999 "Be an Advocate!" speech included a story about a legislator saying she changed her vote since her office was deluged with calls. When asked how many calls she received, she told our lobbyist, "Five." Five is no longer a deluge—maybe not even a trickle. Gone are the days when ginning up a handful of calls could cause someone to rethink their vote. Gone is the default of calling a press conference to get attention to an issue.

Given the vitriol that too often passes for public discourse, more conversation is moving out of the public square and into quieter spaces. Stakeholder meetings are becoming an increasingly popular way for policymakers to understand more about priorities. Fortunately, NCPeds' decades of advocacy, coupled with ever-present lobbyists and strong partners like the NC Medical Society, NC Academy of Family Physicians, and NC Child, mean that we often get a seat at the table to talk about child health issues.

Our members are an invaluable resource here. A quiet call from a pediatrician friend talking through the potential impact of a proposal can mean far more than the best-worded tweet or packed room press conference or hearing. As many kindergarten teachers have demonstrated, the way to cut through the noise sometimes is an effective whisper. But that only works when you are in the room.

Legislative advocacy is not the only type of advocacy: The law and underlying budget clearly matter, but how that law gets implemented also has a huge impact on how families can actually benefit. For example, in 2014, the General Assembly mandated moving to multiple managed care plans for Medicaid through contracts with commercial carriers and required the NC Department of Health and Human Services (NCDHHS) to hone the details.

Knowing that Medicaid primarily serves children (70 percent), NCPeds was deeply engaged in transforming to managed care for Medicaid. Once it became apparent this was a fait accompli at the legislative level, we worked to assure statutory protections on a uniform preferred drug list, streamlined credentialing, strong care-management, and plan-assignment algorithms that kept siblings together in a practice, while assuring existing protections for patients and practices also applied to the new plans.

Once the new law passed, we also worked closely with the department to inform the development of policies and assure that the impact on children remained a top consideration. We reviewed thousands of pages of proposals, wrote more than forty

> Working together to keep a sustained and strategic focus on child health has made an important difference for families in NC.

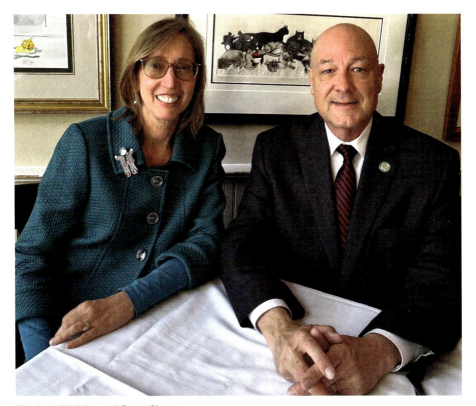

**Elizabeth Hudgins and Steve Shore**

sets of comments, and had three standing monthly meetings with the department. Our leadership also drove to Washington, DC, to meet with Centers for Medicare and Medicaid (CMS) to discuss the proposed waiver moving NC to managed care for Medicaid.

Initially, the NCDHHS policy assigned newborns to the same health plans as the mothers. Pediatricians realized the risk of this policy. A good health plan for pregnant women may not be the best plan for babies—indeed it was possible that a pediatric office may not contract at all with a PHP (Prepaid Health Plan) in which local mothers are enrolled for ob-gyn care. At the same time, rounding in the newborn nursery was already time-consuming, and some practices no longer offered this service. NCPeds was deeply concerned that this administrative policy would create a barrier to community pediatric practices or hospitals providing this important service, as well as providing other care during the critical early months. (Our earlier advocacy on newborn eligibility showed that even when the practice actively encouraged and welcomed newborn visits before the family received their Medicaid card, some families were reluctant to come in for well-child or even sick visits.) We worked with the department to inform changes to the policy so that for the first ninety days after birth, a provider will be paid at in-network rates by all plans to minimize disruption in care. Also, the family will have a Medicaid insurance card that works and can feel comfortable accessing care.

By understanding what babies and their families need, and being part of the discussion, pediatricians were able to help craft policies likely to improve maternal and child health. NCPeds works with partners from several state agencies and commissions on multiple issues to assure optimal outcomes for children, families, and child health professionals. Dozens of pediatricians serve on committees and task forces, bringing a vital child health perspective to how policies, statutes, and rules work for children and families. Examples range from the Commission on Children and Youth with Special Health Care Needs, to the board for the NC Partnership for Children, to the physician advisory group for Medicaid, and the staff for the five different prepaid health plans that now operate Medicaid.

The next step is becoming more intentional in addressing the issues of race, equity, and inclusion. NCPeds has an amazing history of successful advocacy for some of the most vulnerable children in NC—whether we are talking about kids who have been abused and neglected, are low-income and may struggle to access health care, or are medically fragile. But research and life increasingly demonstrate that a rising tide does not lift all boats. At NCPeds, we have become much more intentional in the past several years about assuring that our board and committees are more diverse; our education sessions come from speakers of different races and ethnicities, and we track more internal data on race and ethnicity. We also need to apply this intentionality to our policy work. One of our "family" stories is that when considering drugs for the preferred drug list, liquids were left off the formulary. Because Dr. Theresa Flynn was there to participate in the decision-making in Raleigh and noted that six-month-olds could not swallow tablets, liquids were added.

This story speaks to the reality that even well-meaning and well-informed people may need help understanding multiple aspects of an issue. For a long time, we have lifted up the need for having a child focused perspective in policy conversations. If we want to truly close racial gaps in health care and child outcomes, we need to turn our sustained and strategic lens specifically to addressing racial inequities—one better and intentional policy step at a time.

*Editor's note: Elizabeth Hudgins came highly recommended to the NCPeds leadership because of her service as legislative coordinator for NC Child, the leading child advocacy organization in the state, and her tenure as executive director of the NC Child Fatality Task Force, the legislative entity that develops child-friendly proposals for the General Assembly. At the task force, she worked with Chairpersons Dr. Peter Morris (former president of NCPeds) and Tom Vitaglione (long-term administrator in the NC Division of Maternal and Child Health and senior fellow at NC Child).*

# Part III

# Comprehensive Approach to Advocacy

# The Evolution of North Carolina's Newborn Metabolic Screening Program

by Bob Schwartz, MD, FAAP; Tom Vitaglione, MPH; Rebecca Buckley, MD, FAAP; John Rusher, JD, MD, FAAP

Phenylketonuria (PKU) screening was introduced on a voluntary basis in the early 1960s. Pediatricians statewide influenced their hospitals to adopt PKU screening, and it became universal in 1966, even though there was no statute requiring testing.

In the late 1970s it became feasible to test for congenital hypothyroidism. A bill was introduced to provide funding for the test, as well as to adopt a newborn screening statute that would become the basis for the future of such testing in North Carolina (NC). NCPed's support for the bill led to its passage. In the early 1990s, tandem mass spectrophotometry became available, which would allow for the testing of many more conditions. However, this new technology was very expensive. A metabolic screening laboratory in another state with experience in this technology offered to do the mass spectrophotometry screening testing in our state, and a contract was signed.

After studying the proposal, we found that the new plan would be offered to NC hospitals at a charge. Babies born in hospitals that could afford to pay for the testing would receive the expanded testing, but babies born in hospitals in less affluent areas might not, which would create a two-tier system. This information was presented to the executive committee of NCPeds, and a decision was made to strongly oppose this plan. The contract with the outside laboratory was canceled, and NCPeds helped convince our state government to provide financial support to buy the initial mass spectrophotometry machine. The funding was available in the Maternal and Child Health Block Grant federal allocation. However, we needed an experienced research laboratory to do quality control testing for our first year. Our state laboratory signed an agreement for quality control testing with the same laboratory that made the original offer at a significantly reduced cost. Within a few years, we were able to obtain funding for a second mass spectrophotometry machine.

Finally, NCPeds was influential in convincing the state to follow the standards of the Recommended Uniform Screening Panel. Following those recommendations, NC now screens for almost forty conditions. This example shows the effectiveness of well-organized advocacy efforts by pediatricians working with state professionals for the benefit of infants and children.

In 2015, NCPeds took advantage of an opportunity to convince the legislature to fund the addition of Severe Combined Immune Deficiency (SCID, or "bubble boy disease") to the newborn screening agenda. The newborn screening advisory committee recommended the state fund SCID screening in 2011, but the approximately $500,000 of continuation funding was not approved by legislators. Early in the general session of 2015, Senator Jeffrey Tarte, husband of a pediatrician, introduced a bill to eliminate the religious exemption clause from the childhood immunization statutes, if all babies born in the state could be screened for immune deficiency before the administration of vaccines recommended at two months of age. When the senator received vociferous opposition from the anti-vaccine community, he withdrew the bill. Very quickly, NCPeds convinced legislators to support funding for SCID screening of all babies so that if, in the future, a similar religious exemption bill could be introduced, we already would be screening all babies for immune deficiency well before two months of age. Rebecca Buckley, MD, FAAP, professor of pediatrics and immunology at Duke University School of Medicine, came to Raleigh along with the mother of Carlie Nugent, a baby who had died with SCID but who very well may have lived had she been identified at birth and offered bone marrow transplantation. Duke University has performed the most bone marrow transplants for SCID of any medical center in the world, and Dr. Buckley has been the leader of those efforts. Dr. Buckley also presented very compelling cost-effectiveness data to support SCID screening of all newborns. They convinced the legislature to appropriate the $466,000 in continuation funding so that NC could be added to the list of states that screen all newborns for SCID.

A summary from Dr. Buckley about convincing the legislature to fund SCID screening of all newborns: " . . . I must give the most credit to the wonderfully persuasive speech the mother of a SCID baby who died made. (Dr. Buckley had recruited the mother to come with her to the legislature to testify for our proposal.) Her infant died from overwhelming infections before she could be saved by a transplant. The mother also pointed out to the legislators that the amount one would spend

**INITIATION OF NEWBORN SCREENING TESTS IN NORTH CAROLINA**

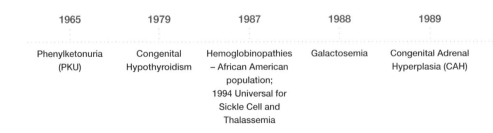

| 1965 | 1979 | 1987 | 1988 | 1989 |
|------|------|------|------|------|
| Phenylketonuria (PKU) | Congenital Hypothyroidism | Hemoglobinopathies – African American population; 1994 Universal for Sickle Cell and Thalassemia | Galactosemia | Congenital Adrenal Hyperplasia (CAH) |

on a nice lunch would cover the cost of screening one newborn for SCID. The response from the legislators was "Why did this take so long to pass—a no-brainer?" I also presented comparative data on how much more it costs Medicaid to pay for a hospitalized sick SCID baby than for one transplanted without infection.

# Child Abuse and Neglect: Creating a High-Quality System

by Sara Sinal, MD, FAAP; Molly Curtin Berkoff, MD, FAAP; V. Denise Everett, MD, FAAP

When we talk to our national peers, we are often asked, "How did you do that in North Carolina?" The answer is simple: "We have the NC Pediatric Society (NCPeds)!" With support from NCPeds, the ability to improve access to care for suspected victims of child maltreatment and children in foster care have improved. We are a national leader because of our efforts.

In the early 1970s when child abuse experts and centers were coming of age, a child abuse committee was established by NCPeds. Initially, the achievements were NCPeds' serious support of this work, trying to establish standards of practice (slide reviews by teleconference), developing multidisciplinary relationships, discussion of funding issues, and ongoing help in medico-legal testimony in courts in child abuse cases.

Child maltreatment has not only been seen as a national crisis over the years, but also a significant challenge throughout the state of North Carolina. The Committee on Child Abuse & Neglect (CCAN) was the largest committee of NCPeds during during the term of V. Denise Everett, MD, FAAP, as chair (1988–2010), and its success can be attributed to the highly dedicated pediatricians specializing in child

| pilot 1997, permanent 1999 | 2004 | 2009 | 2017 | 2021 |
|---|---|---|---|---|
| Tandem Mass Spectrometry (MS/MS) - Amino Acid, Organic Acid, Fatty Acid Oxidation Disorders | Biotinidase Deficiency | Cystic Fibrosis | Severe Combined Immunodeficiency (SCID) | Spinal Muscular Atrophy (SMA) |

abuse evaluation across the state, as well as numerous state agencies and child advocacy organizations who have collaborated with CCAN over the years.

When Dr. Everett joined CCAN in 1987, the committee consisted of just a few pediatricians who specialized in the evaluation of child abuse. Upon becoming chair of CCAN in 1988, Dr. Everett began inviting state agencies to attend meetings because the topics were expanding from the complexities of the child abuse evaluation and treatment process to much broader issues. These included billing and compensation (due to individual child abuse programs struggling financially, given the time involved in not only conducting child abuse evaluations, but the time involved subsequent to the evaluation process), writing reports, communicating with affiliated agencies, making referrals to mental health, and testimony, as needed, in court. Dr. Everett spearheaded the effort to secure Current Procedural Terminology (CPT) coding specifically for child abuse through the American Medical Association.

As the topics for discussion continued to expand, Dr. Everett felt the need to begin seeking representation from not only state agencies, but also child advocacy organizations. Within a few years, organizations were asking to join CCAN.

Collaborations were established between the committee and many state agencies and organizations, including: NC Child Medical Evaluation Program, NC Division of Social Services, NC Community Child Protection Team, NC Attorney General's Office, NC Guardian ad Litem Program, Child Advocacy Centers of NC, NC Child Fatality Prevention Team, NC Fatality Review Team, NC Coalition Against Sexual Assault, and Prevent Child Abuse NC. Without the input and collaboration from these organizations' nurses, social workers, lawyers, and administrators, the achievements of the committee would not have been possible.

Through the collaboration of all of these agencies and organizations, along with the support of NCPeds, CCAN was able to accomplish many successes, such as providing statewide guidelines on evaluation and treatment of child maltreatment for pediatricians and sexual assault nurse examiners (SANEs). Other positive outcomes included legislative changes, court testimony advances, addressing both the physical and mental health trauma of child maltreatment, and improving the welfare and safety of children in North Carolina.

During Dr. Everett's tenure as chair, the CCAN continued to be the central contact point in the state for addressing issues surrounding child maltreatment.

NCPeds has been a staunch supporter of the NC Child Medical Evaluation Program (CMEP). This program assists with access to comprehensive medical assessments of children who are being investigated by child protective services for child maltreatment. All components of the medical evaluation, including laboratory studies and radiology studies, are offered at no cost to the family. The 1976–1977 founding of this program by the state's chief medical examiner, Dr. Page Hudson, and the chief of community pediatrics at UNC, Dr. Frank Loda, was supported from the beginning by NCPeds with a goal of identifying providers in every county in the state who would provide expert evaluations. The program also has been well-supported by the practicing physicians in the state; in a survey of pediatricians about their court experiences published in 2006, three-fourths of the state's private pediatricians reported having been, or still being part of, the CMEP program. There has always been time during open forums and in the exhibit hall space at the NCPeds annual meeting so that the CMEP can educate and recruit pediatricians, provide updates in the evaluation and management of maltreatment in the medical setting, and update aspects of Child Protective Services (CPS) policy that impact medical providers. The NCPeds Committee on Child Abuse provided continuing advice and guidance to this program and, over the years, identified areas of need. These areas include improving the understanding of etiologies of abusive head trauma and developing mechanisms for mental health evaluations to complement assessments and improve recommendations.

*Through the collaboration of all of these agencies and organizations, along with the support of NCPeds, CCAN was able to accomplish many successes.*

NCPeds was called upon at several critical junctures to provide support for augmenting and maintaining the program. In the late 1980s, with the recognition that evaluation of child sexual abuse had become more specialized and complex, the society went to bat at the legislature to support resources for enhancing child interviews and the use of instrumentation such as colposcopy; the legislature responded favorably. At that time, it was documented that for the previous five years, medical provider retention and recruitment had been difficult. Again, reimbursement and time had become limitations in assuring children had access to the most expert assessments.

With support from NCPeds, NC CMEP enacted a specific state policy, supported by NC Division of Social Services and NC Medicaid, to provide enhanced payment for providers. Now with support from NCPeds, NC CMEP can provide quality oversight of all outpatient medical consultations for NC Division of Social Services (more than 4,000/annually).

Without NCPeds, this new policy and enhanced payment would not have been attainable. To make the changes possible, the NCPeds executive director developed the strategy and provided opportunities for pediatrician advocates to speak in front of key legislators and leaders of the Department of Health and Human Services. We have had amazing support from the executive directors of NCPeds, Steve Shore, MSW, (2000-2015) and Elizabeth Hudgins, MSS (2015-present).

In recent years, the CCAN has broadened its agenda and engaged in the following additional successful campaigns:

> 1. With approval from the NC Hospital Association and the NC College of Emergency Physicians, the CCAN developed emergency department guidelines for child physical abuse evaluations and emergency department guidelines for child sexual abuse evaluations. These were distributed to emergency departments statewide. The guidelines have been updated over time with the latest update occurring in 2015.

> 2. In collaboration with the child abuse committee and the NC Forensic Nurses Association, guidelines for sexual assault nurse examiners in performing pediatric examinations were formulated.

> 3. Guidelines also were created for the evaluation of medical child abuse (Munchausen syndrome by proxy).

Several members of the committee expressed concern about sexual exploitation of children in advertising. This resulted in a Let Kids Be Kids campaign.

The issue of children being left alone—when is it acceptable and when is it considered neglect—was discussed at a number of meetings. A pamphlet was published, providing guidance to parents as to when it was safe to leave children home alone. Suggestions for improving safety for children when alone also were provided. These were the Home Safe Series, "Is Your Child Ready to Stay Home Alone?"

In early 2010, several pediatrician members of the committee had been involved in the treatment of three horrendous physical abuse and neglect cases in children who were being homeschooled. Two of these cases resulted in the death of the child. In addition, there was another case of severe and repeated sexual abuse of a homeschooled child. The issues of homeschooling and abuse were investigated at length. The investigation documented the monitoring of homeschools in NC by the NC DNPE (Department of Non-Public Education). The CCAN collaborated with one of three homeschool associations in NC that offer support to homeschool families. The outcome was a publication outlining the homeschool situation in NC, and a list of recommendations for pediatricians who may have homeschooled children in their practices. Speakers were provided to the homeschool parents annual meeting regarding parents' ability to recognize and report abuse if they suspect it in a homeschool family.

Subsequent committee chairs have been Dr. Meggan Goodpasture (2010–2017) and Dr. Stacy Thomas (2018–present).

NCPeds has been instrumental in
ensuring excellent access to high quality
care for NC's most vulnerable children.

In 2014, Dr. Cindy Brown introduced pediatricians in the committee to a "No Hit Policy." Drs. Goodpasture and Brown agreed to pilot this in their clinics with the idea encouraging a statewide initiative.

In 2015 Dr. Aditee Narayan developed a track within the committee for trainee membership to include medical students, residents, and fellows. Many learners have taken advantage of the membership. The goals were increasing interest in the field of child abuse and neglect and modeling advocacy.

In 2017, the committee took a highly active role in supporting Dr. Molly Berkoff and the child medical evaluation program in successful efforts to increase reimbursement for child abuse and neglect evaluations in the state of NC.

In 2019, a subcommittee developed guidelines for evaluation of physical abuse in children's advocacy centers that were distributed to these centers.

\*\*\*

In 2020, the committee developed a summary of suggestions for pediatricians in NC for dealing with child abuse concerns during the pandemic: *Managing Child Abuse Concerns During the COVID-19 Pandemic – Thoughts from the Committee on Child Abuse and Neglect. This was distributed through NCPeds.*

In 2021, several members of the committee helped update the medical section of the North Carolina Conference of District Attorneys' Child Maltreatment Guidelines for Prosecutors.

Prior to NCPeds taking the lead on the Fostering Health initiative (see *Redesigning Foster Care*), it was challenging for most general pediatricians and other child health professionals to understand issues regarding consent, ensuring prompt access to care, and even understanding key elements of the medical history relevant to the abuse and neglect of foster children. As a result, the care of children was suboptimal.

In recent years, NCPeds' actions have resulted in significant improvements in care. They have not only created a free, readily accessible library of tools and educational materials, they have worked to create a multidisciplinary system that ensures easy and timely access to care as well as robust case management for children. This ensures that child welfare workers and foster families have a clear understanding of their children's diagnoses, medications, and other treatment needs. In summary, the NCPeds has been instrumental in ensuring excellent access to high quality care for NC's most vulnerable children.[1]

## Abolishing Corporal Punishment in North Carolina's Public Schools

by Tom Vitaglione, MPH

Corporal punishment has been used in North Carolina's public schools since colonial times. It was not until the mid-1980s, however, that the practice was formally allowed by statute, and school personnel were given immunity from prosecution unless it could be proven that a student was seriously injured intentionally. The state's corporal punishment statute is considered to be the most grisly of all statutes affecting children.

> In all communities, pediatricians have special places of respect among families and community leaders.

The formal statute provided the focus for a statewide campaign to ban the practice. The initial focus was on the legislature itself, in hopes of achieving a statewide ban. An advocacy coalition grew around this objective, and the NC Pediatric Society (NCPeds) was a prominent member. The "gravitas" of the society and its members provided credibility to the campaign.

It is not happenstance that the initial and current legislative champions to ban corporal punishment come from the Asheville area, where Dr. Olson Huff, a respected member of the community, effectively recruited them to the cause. Despite several valiant attempts over the years, the legislature still remains reluctant to adopt a statewide ban, even though thirty-one states have now done so.

The statute did say that local school districts had the authority to ban the practice locally. Given the slim chances of a statewide ban, it became evident that we needed to undertake the arduous task of approaching each of the 115 local school districts. And, once again, the role of pediatricians became critical.

[1.] Goodpasture, Meggan, V. D. Everett, Martha Gagliano, Aditee P. Narayan, and Sara Sinal. "Invisible Children." *North Carolina Medical Journal* 74, no. 1 (2013): 90-94.

In all communities, pediatricians have special places of respect among families and community leaders. Pediatricians have become the best messengers regarding the negative effects of corporal punishment and the need to ban the practice in schools.

In a number of school districts, a pediatrician was a member of the district board. Almost invariably, these became the first districts to ban the practice. In other districts, pediatricians were identified and asked to help lead the local advocacy efforts. Once again, the pediatric voice carried the day in district after district. And in 2018, the last of the 115 districts banned corporal punishment!

This is a prominent example of the role that North Carolina's pediatricians continue to play in improving the health and well-being of our children.

# Gun Violence: A Pediatric Problem That Requires Multidisciplinary Advocacy

by Dave Tayloe Jr., MD, FAAP

In 1983, John Niblock and friends established the NC Child Advocacy Institute, now known as NC Child. It is the leading force in child advocacy in our state today. Dr. Frank Gearing, a community pediatrician in Wilson and member of the executive committee of NCPeds, joined the board of the institute in 1983, assuring collaboration of the two organizations going forward. Dr. Gearing worked with the institute to establish a telephone tree, whereby pediatricians and members of the institute were linked to every one of the 170 legislators in the NC General Assembly.

Frank and I were both elected to the NC Peds Executive Committee in 1983, and we became close friends. When I became seriously involved in promoting vaccine liability legislation in 1985 (see *Big Dave: Visionary Leader*), I worked closely with Frank to assure that the legislative telephone tree was working effectively. The key contact system enabled us to efficiently involve community and academic pediatricians, along with members of the institute, in our lobbying efforts around vaccine liability.

At the invitation of Dr. Gearing, John Niblock began attending the NCPeds Liaison Committee meetings and was often given time in the programs to update attendees on the activities of the institute. When I became chair of the NCPeds Committee on Legislation, I invited John to co-host legislative symposia with NCPeds on the Saturdays when the institute conducted its annual black-tie dinner dance/fundraiser. This was called the "Gala," and was held at a hotel in the Triangle region of Raleigh-Durham-Chapel Hill.

John and I would select topics for the symposia, and we would recruit speakers. Then we shared the facilitator role for the afternoon sessions that occurred in the on the same day and at the same hotel where the gala would take place that night.

The most memorable legislative symposium occurred on January 30, 1993, in Durham, and was entitled, "Guns and Schools in North Carolina." NCPeds conducted its liaison committee meeting in the morning before the legislative symposium scheduled for the afternoon, with the gala to follow that night. There were seventy-eight pediatricians and lay child advocates at the liaison committee meeting, and 150 attendees for the "Guns and Schools" program. Speakers included the executive director of the leading child advocacy group in Charlotte, an emergency medicine pediatrician from Chicago representing the American Academy of Pediatrics, a district court judge, the lobbyist for NCPeds, and two influential state legislators—one from the Senate and one from the House of Representatives. There were leaders from the Durham community in attendance who made comments that brought the problems of guns and schools to life for attendees.

Tom Vitaglione, MPH (see *The Growth of Collaboration*), participated in the symposium as an administrator in the Department of Health and Human Services and referred to the event as a "watershed moment" when leaders from multiple backgrounds and organizations came together to focus on the problems of gun violence, especially as they affect school-aged children.

Following the event, gun responsibility legislation was quietly introduced and ushered successfully through the statute-making process to become law, making gun owners responsible for injuries and death when minors obtained guns and inflicted harm upon themselves or others (see *Stepping Up Our Advocacy: Hiring an Experienced Lobbyist*).

# Creating a User-Friendly Kindergarten Health Assessment

by R.M. (Mac) Herring Jr., MD, FAAP

Prior to 1985, there was no uniform requirement or mechanism for health care personnel to transmit a health and developmental assessment to schools for children entering kindergarten in our state. There was a hodgepodge array of requirements varying from local education agencies (LEAs) and even from school to school within an LEA.

Few LEAs required anything at all and most that did documented only height and weight. In fact, there was no uniform assessment of NC children after early infancy or maybe even after their nursery stay. Note that prior to 1975–1977, the developmental evaluation centers (DECs) provided a limited number of screens for children with developmental problems, but in 1978 the emphasis of the DECs was transferred to infant screening in the high priority infant screening program.

In the 1980s, there developed a growing concern about this lack of preschool assessment within the state among the Department of Public Instruction (DPI), Division of Health Services (DHS) and the pediatric community. This culminated in the formation of a committee in 1983 to study the feasibility of kindergarten screening. Dr. Mac Herring was appointed to this committee along with personnel from DPI, DHS, and other members of the private sector. Other NCPeds members on the committee included Drs. Tom Frothingham, Jonnie McLeod, Raymond Sturner, Ann Wolfe, Jimmy Rhyne, and Tom Vitaglione, MPH. This committee expressed recognition of the positive potential for a kindergarten health assessment to provide health and educational advantages, and even developed an initial assessment form. This assessment form was transmitted for review and comment to several NCPeds members, including Drs. Henry Hawthorne, David Tayloe Sr., Robert Schwartz, Keith Thompson, Wes Garbee, and Floyd Denny (eminent chairperson of pediatrics at UNC). Dr. Herring gathered comments and constructive criticism from these individuals and presented them to our committee for revisions to the assessment form. The committee spent considerable time discussing and reviewing the suggestions and revising the form which was then presented along with the committee report to Dr. Ron Levine, director of DHS, and Mr. Ted Drain, director of exceptional children, DPI.

This committee report, which recommended a mandatory kindergarten health assessment, received a favorable response from Dr. Levine and Mr. Drain in October 1984. The NCPeds Liaison Committee enthusiastically supported this recommendation for pre-kindergarten screening in September 1984, as did the general membership of NCPeds and NC Medical Society. NCPeds voiced the opinion that such a health assessment was important to identify major medical and/or developmental problems that might interfere with the educational process or adaptation to the classroom. DPI and medical care providers could then work together to provide continuity of services, and the data gathered would enable more careful health care and educational planning for the future.

This background effort culminated in the introduction of Senate Bill 293, An Act to Require Health Assessments for Kindergarten Children in the Public Schools, by Senator Laura Tally in 1985. This bill did receive a favorable report from the education committee but died in the Senate appropriations committee. Strategy was developed between Dr. Jimmy Rhyne, the pediatric legislative committee, and Henry Jones, our NCPeds lobbyist, to resurrect this bill in the 1986 legislative session. There were some legislative concerns about costs. The legislature was reassured that the development of a form had been completed and there would be no additional cost. There was concern about increased Medicaid expenditure to treat identified problems, and the bill was rewritten in 1986 to provide funds to DPI for developmental screening.

There was some misunderstanding in July 1986 that NC pediatricians would provide these screens at no cost for low-income non-Medicaid patients. Henry Jones helped clarify this misunderstanding with the legislature as health department directors stated they could meet the needs of these patients. Fortunately, with the efforts of individual members of our society contacting their legislators, and Mr. Henry Jones lobbying on our behalf and other concerned parties, this Senate Bill 293 did pass in 1986 to become effective July 1, 1987.

Dr. Herring was appointed to a committee to review the assessment form along with Dr. Jimmy Rhyne, Dr. Ray Sturner, and Dr. Tom Frothingham. Again, Dr. Herring insisted that our efforts be reviewed by community pediatricians, including Drs. Steve Edwards, Dave Tayloe Jr., Robert Schwartz, George Prince, Wes Garbee, Henry Hawthorne, Dave Williams, Keith Thompson, Tom McCutchen, Mike Dennis, and Wally Brown. Utilizing their comments, revisions were completed, and a new form was approved in 1990.

Some local health departments initially resisted being involved in these assessments. Fortunately, Dr. Thad Wester, pediatrician, and member of the pediatric liaison committee, was president of the NC Health Directors Association in 1987. He was instrumental in obtaining the cooperation of all local health departments to participate in this screening process.

As the program was rolled out over the next couple of years, problems and concerns over the assessment form arose, and revisions were made with input to DPI from the NCPeds Liaison Committee and community pediatricians. A new form was adopted in 1990. There was still another revision to the form in 1996 with DPI listening to our pediatricians attempting to streamline the form to encourage more accurate and complete information.

This law to require health and developmental assessments of children entering kindergarten in our state has persisted to this time. Administrators in the Department of Health and Human Services continue to meet regularly with representatives of NCPeds, NC Academy of Family Physicians, school nurses, and administrators from the Department of Public Instruction to assure the form is user-friendly for families, pediatricians, and school staff. Changes require action by the General Assembly.

In 2015, a revised form was approved so that any child, regardless of grade level, entering a given public school district (LEA) for the first time, would be required to have the equivalent of the kindergarten health assessment during the first thirty days of matriculation. There is some concern that this new form is not as detail-oriented as it needs to be to reflect the true health of the entering student. NCPeds leaders will work to improve this form going forward.

This uniform mandate has been of medical and educational benefit to children. It is my belief that the NCPeds, the pediatric liaison committee/open forum; our lobbyist, Henry Jones; and individual pediatricians were instrumental in the passage of this important legislation.

## Pull the Plug on TV Violence

by Kathleen Clarke-Pearson, MD, FAAP

As a North Carolina pediatrician, I am grateful for how the NC Pediatric Society (NCPeds) supported me in starting a three-year Pull the Plug on TV Violence project directed at educating North Carolina families about the negative impacts cartoon and other television depictions of violence have on kids. The year was 1995.

That year, three of my four children, who were all attending Chapel Hill public schools, lost three classmates in gun-associated incidents. One took his life, and the other two students were victims of accidental shootings. The community was overwhelmed with grief about these nonsensical deaths. Our local parent teacher association (PTA) rallied and held a Pull The Plug on TV Violence event on Memorial Day dedicated to the three kids who died. Information was provided to all school families about how glamorized TV violence contributes to children's decisions to play with guns.

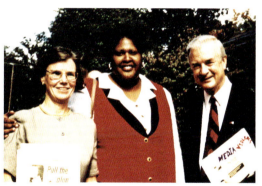

Left to Right: Dr. Kathleen Clarke-Pearson with Sheila Bazemore and Governor James B. Hunt, promoting "Pull the Plug"

I was so concerned about a lot of children watching gratuitous violence on television that I contacted our NCPeds president, Dave Tayloe Jr., and asked him to have the society prioritize exposure to TV violence and its negative impact on kids. He responded quickly with a letter of support, a $5,000 check, and the names of three strong child advocates who would soon join hands with me in forming the NC Pull the Plug on TV Violence Coalition.

This was a three-year project supported by Governor James Hunt. We distributed pamphlets and bumper stickers to every public elementary school in every NC county, targeting kindergarten to third grade students and providing facts about the importance of parental supervision of TV use. Our coalition grew to number thirty-four partners including the NC Parent Teacher Association, Prevend Child Abuse NC, NC Department of Health and Human Services, and NC Child (formerly the NC Child Advocacy Institute). Dr. Olson Huff, who followed in Dr. Tayloe Jr.'s footsteps at the helm of NCPeds, provided me with much sound advice about how to strengthen the coalition. My NCPeds colleagues, who lived in various counties, embraced the project and supported our efforts to distribute the pamphlets and bumper stickers around the state. I remain very grateful for the terrific support that NCPeds provided to launch this much-needed child advocacy project!

## Into the Mouths of Babes: A Collaborative Solution for Improving Children's Oral Health

by Emily Horney, MHA, RDH; Olson Huff, MD, FAAP; Martha Ann Keels, DDS, PhD; Rebecca King, DDS, MPH; Steve Shore, MSW; Dave Tayloe Jr., MD, FAAP

During the 1990s, research involving primary care medical—not dental—professionals applying fluoride varnish to the teeth of at-risk preschool children showed significant reductions in early dental caries. A proposal to conduct a demonstration project in very rural settings, where children's access to dental professionals was extremely challenging, was formed by an alliance of child health, dental, and medical advocates in the public and private sectors. The goal was to improve the oral health of children in rural areas of Western North Carolina. The intervention included application of fluoride varnish to preschool age children's teeth coupled with a methodical but practical oral health examination, and education about good oral health habits.

Dr. James Bawden, pediatric dentist at the University of North Carolina School of Dentistry and dean of the school for eight years, was a world-renowned dental researcher. Dr. Bawden conducted extensive studies in the areas of enamel formation and uptake of fluoride varnish into tooth enamel. Based on his work and the results of dental researchers in Japan and Sweden, he led the effort from 1995–2001 to create, fund, and implement an oral health initiative called Smart Smiles in a nine-county area of Western North Carolina. Meetings involved the UNC School of Dentistry; NC Oral Health Section staff based in the NC Department of Health and Human Services (DHHS); the NC Partnership for Children (Smart Start)[2]; and personnel from the Ruth and Billy Graham Children's Health Center in Asheville. The results included the development of protocols for primary care practice-based application of fluoride varnish to children's teeth as an evidence-based intervention.

---

[2.] Smart Start is the kindergarten-readiness initiative of state government, focused on improving access and quality in child day care, that was established during the 1990s by Governor Jim Hunt and the state legislature. All preschool children in NC are eligible for services through local Smart Start organizations that are operating in most of the one hundred counties.

# Significant changes in the oral health care for our young patients occurred because North Carolina child advocates made it happen!

The roll-out of an oral health pilot project in Western North Carolina was a result of several factors:

1. Dr. Bawden was front and center with the scientific evidence to do it;

2. The steering committee obtained a $1 million dollar grant from the Appalachian Regional Commission (ARC) to fund the demonstration effort;

3. Monica Teutsch, who managed the Graham Health Center's dental program, along with Doug Sailor of the Toe River Health District office in Burnsville (also affiliated with the Graham Center), provided critical support efforts to assure efficient implementation of the pilot protocols.

*Dr. Olson Huff comments: I remember that some of the meetings we had with Dr. Bawden and the dental hygienists took place in my wife Marilyn's training center in Black Mountain, next to the Swannanoa River! As Dr. Bawden and Ms. Teutsch were getting the dental varnish project going, I was engaging in a major commitment to entice dentists to take care of indigent children, including those on Medicaid. A rather interesting part of this was the resistance of the American Academy of Pediatrics (AAP) executive director to change the periodicity schedule for when pediatricians should perform oral health exams on children! We changed that standard from age three to age one! The bottom line of all this, however, is that significant changes in the oral health care for our young patients occurred because North Carolina child advocates made it happen!*

Financial payment for incorporating the Smart Smiles protocols by primary care providers became a significant barrier. An NC Institute of Medicine Advisory Committee partnered with Smart Smiles leaders, and in 1999, recommended that the Division of Medical Assistance develop a new service delivery package, claims filing, and payment method, utilizing Current Dental Terminology (CDT) codes to reimburse for early caries screening, education, and administration of fluoride varnish provided by physicians and physician extenders to children between the ages of nine and thirty-six months.

In the fall of 1999, meetings were conducted with the program director and dental director of NC Medicaid in the Department of Health and Human Services (DHHS), the president of NCPeds, the president of the NC Academy of Family Physicians, faculty members from the University of North Carolina Chapel Hill School of Dentistry, and dental professionals in the Oral Health Section of DHHS. The goal was to develop a strategy for statewide implementation. The plan—named "Into the Mouths of Babes" and abbreviated as IMB—was based on a three-part preventive package with Medicaid payment. Primary care providers would make a visual examination of the mouth and teeth based on existing child health primary care procedures, provide age-appropriate dental education and counseling for parents or caregivers, and apply the fluoride varnish.

Based on the success of the Western North Carolina pilot project, with evaluation results tabulated by the Oral Health Section and University of North Carolina dental researchers, Dr. Bawden persuaded NC Medicaid to pay primary care health professionals an equitable fee to incorporate the three-part oral health agenda into child health office encounters. Successive NC Medicaid Dental Directors Betty King-Sutton, DMD, and Mark Casey, DDS, MPH, provided strong support for launching and developing IMB statewide.

Traditionally, primary care health professionals were expected to do comprehensive oral health examinations, so there would be no extra payment for this service. For educating the families about evidence-based oral health care in the home and applying fluoride varnish to all teeth, providers were able to file claims utilizing two CDT codes for payment by Medicaid—one for providing education and one for applying the fluoride varnish to all teeth.

Dr. Bawden met with the leadership of NCPeds, and made a presentation during an open forum meeting of the society to gain support of the pediatricians for the IMB Program. Kelly Close, RDH, MPA, a dental hygienist, was hired using IMB grant funds from Medicaid and state appropriations to the DHHS Oral Health Section budget to coordinate IMB implementation. She was provided office space by NCPeds in January 2001 when the society offices were temporarily located in the office building of the NC Academy of Family Physicians in Raleigh. This arrangement proved to be helpful in coordinating the training efforts aimed at both family physicians and pediatricians. Close began preparing a comprehensive toolkit for physicians that included the complete evidence-based background for the intervention along with information about how to conduct the office procedure and how to code and bill Medicaid for the service.

Several pediatricians became leaders and mentors in the effort to convince pediatricians to participate in the IMB Program. Dr. Olson Huff, past-president of NCPeds, assisted Dr. Bawden and administrators in the DHHS Oral Health Section

# Several pediatricians became leaders and mentors in the effort to convince pediatricians to participate in the IMB Program.

in advocating that pediatricians incorporate IMB procedures into their practices. Dr. Huff served as the American Academy of Pediatrics' Oral Health Champion for North Carolina. Dr. Joe Ponzi, pediatrician in Goldsboro, and Dr. Graham Barden III, pediatrician in New Bern, traveled to other practices to demonstrate to pediatric practitioners the ease with which the IMB agenda could be implemented during routine office encounters and to convince the pediatricians that they would be paid fairly for adding the program to their practice agendas. They appeared in a well-used video that included Dr. Bawden's didactic presentation on the dental science behind the intervention, with pediatricians demonstrating how to conduct the procedure.

The state's five pediatric residency programs also adopted the IMB program as a module to be incorporated into pediatric residency education. Duke Pediatrics Primary Care was the first academic clinic to adopt the IMB program in the state. It was helpful that the division chief of Pediatric Primary Care at Duke was Dr. Dennis Clements, whose wife, Dr. Martha Ann Keels, is a pediatric dentist. Dr. Keels was one of the pioneers of the Section of Oral Health at the AAP, and helped to promote the IMB program across the country, modeling the NC innovative initiative. Along with other national pediatric and pediatric dental leaders, Dr. Keels co-authored several AAP Oral Health policy statements impacting pediatric oral health worldwide.

Because of these collaborative efforts, most pediatricians, many family physicians, and local health department clinics began to participate in the IMB Program. Dr. R. Gary Rozier, public health dentist, and peers at the UNC School of Public Health were able to document significant reductions in early childhood caries in elementary school children within five-to-ten years of the implementation of the IMB Program.[3,4]

[3] *Arch Pediatr Adolesc Med.* Author manuscript; available in PMC 2015 Oct 19.Published in final edited form as: *Arch Pediatr Adolesc Med.* 2012 Oct; 166(10): 945–951.doi: 10.1001/archpediatrics.2012.797 Authors: Martha Ann Keels, Rebecca King, Gary Rozier, Emily Horney) PMCID: PMC4610377NIHMSID (Authors: Kelly Close, Olson Huff, Steve Shore, Dave Tayloe Jr.,: NIHMS415898,PMID: 22926203

[4] "Cost-Effectiveness of Preventive Oral Health Care in Medical Offices for Young Medicaid Enrollees"Authors: Sally C. Stearns, PhD; R. Gary Rozier, DDS, MPH; Ashley M. Kranz, BA; Bhavna T. Pahel, BDS, MPH, PhD; and Rocio B. Quiñonez, DMD, MS, MPH

# Child and Adolescent Mental Health Reform: Improving Access and Quality

by Jane Meschan Foy, MD, FAAP; Marian Earls, MD, MTS, FAAP; David Horowitz, MD, FAAP

North Carolina began efforts to improve mental health (MH) care for its state employees early in the 1990s within the State Employee Health Plan (SEHP), managed by Blue Cross/Blue Shield of North Carolina (BC/BSNC), then a non-profit corporation. BC/BSNC thought that money could be saved by providing affordable access to outpatient MH services so that patients would be less likely to require long term and very expensive inpatient hospital stays. The SEHP offered parity of MH and physical health benefits and began paying for up to twenty-six outpatient MH encounters per year with very little in the way of patient copays and with referral from a primary care physician (PCP) to an MH specialist of the patient's choice, rather than requiring an MH system gatekeeper and limiting access to a panel of providers. As predicted, implementation within the SEHP resulted in net savings when hospitalizations decreased dramatically as access to outpatient services increased. This outcome was important to the later work of NCPeds because it made state agency administrators less wary of expanding access to MH care.

> Implementation within the SEHP resulted in net savings when hospitalizations decreased dramatically as access to outpatient services increased.

In 1998, elected leaders in NC had little appetite for using the new federally-funded State Child Health Insurance Program (SCHIP) to expand Medicaid. The NCPeds leadership was instrumental in convincing the legislature to choose BC/BSNC as the home for NC Health Choice. NCPeds was not fully aware of the MH reforms that had taken place in the SEHP when SCHIP became a reality; however, fortuitously, pediatrician Dr. Dave Bruton served as secretary of the Department of Health and Human Services (DHHS) at the time and regularly attended the NCPeds Liaison Committee (later renamed Open Forum) meetings, where leaders of state agencies and NCPeds members met to share information and address child health issues. Dr. Bruton was central to the implementation of NC Health Choice and ably represented both the interests of children and the perspectives of pediatricians.

106

NC Health Choice was fashioned after the State Employees Health Plan. Enrollees benefited from the same enlightened policies on parity of mental health and physical health benefits and generous access to outpatient MH services by referral from PCPs. In 1998, pediatricians were appointed to leadership positions on the Physician Advisory Committee for NC Health Choice and the NC Health Choice Commission on Children with Special Needs. NCPeds President Jane Foy convened the Physician Advisory Committee with pediatrician Wally Brown as its chair. Tom Vitaglione, long-term friend of NCPeds and an administrator in the NC Division of Maternal and Child Health, convened the Commission on Children with Special Needs, with NCPeds Past-President Dave Tayloe Jr. as chair. These committee and commission meetings were attended by plan administrators and agency leaders, and gave voice to pediatricians in decision-making about the new plan.

NCPeds led the effort to reform Medicaid's MH program, which at the time consisted of an in-person intake procedure and heavy-handed management by public area MH programs; access only to MH providers within those public programs; little-to-no communication between those providers and primary care physicians; and no payment of primary care physicians (PCPs) for MH services that they or their employees provided. From 1998-2000, NCPeds committee chairs and state agency representatives met first in a public library—conveniently located off one of the state's main interstate routes in Alamance County—then in a conference room around the corner from the Raleigh office of Medicaid Director Dick Peruzzi to develop a position paper and policy recommendations for Medicaid, modeled after those in the SEHP. They were successful in developing and implementing new Medicaid policies that allowed: credentialing of private sector MH providers (outside state government's area MH programs); up to six unmanaged MH visits to the PCP without a definite mental health diagnosis (critical in pediatrics, where the younger the child, the increased likelihood that [s]he does not have a Diagnostic and Statistical Manual of Mental Disorders (DSM) diagnosis; up to twenty-six total unmanaged visits to the PCP or an MH provider of the patient's choice on referral from the PCP; payment of PCPs for their MH services; and "incident to" billing for the services of MH professionals employed by PCPs. These policies opened the door to integration of MH professionals (MHPs) within primary care settings and effective collaboration between PCPs and community-based MHPs.

For details of the mental health advocacy effort, see Appendix for *PEDIATRICS*: Foy, JM, Earls, MF, Horowitz, DA, *Working to Improve Mental Health Services: the North Carolina Advocacy Effort*; 2002 Dec: 110(6): 1232-7.

# Child Development

**by Marian Earls, MD, MTS, FAAP**

NCPeds has an established history of supporting innovation and quality improvement in pediatric health care. An example of this is NCPeds' participation in the Assuring Better Child Health and Development (ABCD) Program.

By 1999, NC Medicaid's Carolina Access model had evolved into a statewide system of physician-directed networks that was implementing the Medicaid program in partnership with the NC Department of Health and Human Services' Division of Medical Assistance and NC Office of Rural Health (ORH). Pediatric leadership figured prominently in the early development of Carolina Access. (see *Whys and Hows of Medicaid*)

When a grant to improve developmental services for young children in Medicaid became available from the Commonwealth Fund, the ORH applied. That the ORH pursued this grant reflects the importance of pediatricians' involvement in Carolina Access. The leaders of the ORH asked me to lead the work of the grant. At the time I was medical director of a large safety net pediatric practice that served 66 percent of the children on Medicaid in Guilford County, and was medical director of the Carolina Access network, Guilford Access Partnership.

From the outset, NCPeds was involved. Steve Shore, executive director of NCPeds, was part of our original workgroup at the ORH. Because of Steve's and the NC Pediatric Society's relationship with the NC Academy of Family Physicians (NCAFP), Greg Griggs, their executive director, sent his representative to the work group. This group, in 2001, became the larger, cross-sector ABCD State Advisory Group that continued to meet quarterly, working on policy and administrative barriers until 2020. That group has now become the steering committee of the Early Well Initiative. NCPeds and NCAFP have continued to participate.

The developmental screening rate in primary care in 1999 was at 12 percent at two- and four-year well visits. The Carolina Access networks in Guilford, Forsyth, and a number of counties in Western North Carolina were the earliest participants. We had multiple statewide, all-day training sessions for practices across the state. We also presented at NCPeds annual meetings and open forums, and at NCAFP annual meetings.

Because of the success of ABCD, in 2004, NC Medicaid policy changed to require screening with a validated screening tool at the six, twelve, eighteen or twenty-four, thirty-six, forty-eight, and sixty-month well-visits. In 2010, the policy changed again to require autism screening at the eighteen- and twenty-four-month visits.

NCPeds' impactful contributions to this work are many: the tradition of convening of state partners, the relationship with Medicaid leadership for decisions about policy affecting children, and the credibility with practices across the state.

By 2015, developmental screening rates were at 90 percent at these visits statewide, for both pediatric and family medicine practices. Autism screening was at 79 percent. Perinatal depression screening training and technical assistance became possible in 2013 through the Children's Health Insurance Program Reauthorization Act (CHIPRA) Quality Demonstration Grant that I led at Community Care of NC (CCNC), the mature statewide physician-directed system of care for Medicaid that evolved from Carolina Access.

By the end of 2019, developmental and autism screening at the visits listed above was at 94 percent, and perinatal depression screening at the one-month visit was at 89 percent statewide, according to data from the EPSDT Profile of CCNC's Quarterly Measures and Feedback. For all these years, North Carolina has led the nation with these rates of screening.

This work has not only been about screening. The intentional cross-sector convening and exchange also helped practices learn how to discuss screening with families, how to refer when there are concerns, and about other valuable community linkages. We reached consensus on statewide referral and feedback forms for Part C (ages 0-3 years) and Part B (ages 3-5 years) Early Intervention Programs mandated by the federal Individuals with Disabilities Education Act (IDEA), and worked on processes for standardized communication among primary care providers, care managers, early intervention specialists, and early childhood education professionals.

NCPeds' impactful contributions to this work are many: the tradition of convening of state partners, the relationship with Medicaid leadership for decisions about policy affecting children, and the credibility with practices across the state.

# Directing State Coalitions

by Steve Shore, MSW

## STATE CHILDREN'S HEALTH INSURANCE (SCHIP)

Responding to the political realities that led to the creation of SCHIP, NCPeds played a significant role in the state-sponsored activities to implement North Carolina's program in October 1998. The establishment of North Carolina's stand-alone SCHIP plan and the role of NCPeds in establishing the framework and principles of this program is the subject of another commentary, *Child Health Insurance Program (CHIP): The North Carolina Experience* by Dave Tayloe Jr., MC, FAAP, Olson Huff, MD, FAAP, and Tom Vitaglione, MPH.

When NC Health Choice (the state's name for SCHIP) opened for enrollment, NCPeds immediately engaged in the education, outreach, and enrollment activities organized by the Divisions of Medical Assistance (DMA), Department of Public Health (DPH), and Department of Social Services (DSS) in the NC Department of Health and Human Services (NCDHHS). At the initiation of NC Health Choice, the NC State Employees Health Plan managed the plan with Blue Cross/Blue Shield of North Carolina as the fiscal intermediary to pay providers. NCPeds President Jane Foy, MD, FAAP, assembled a task force to help troubleshoot problems for all health providers. Wally Brown, MD, FAAP, of Raleigh, chaired the initial NC Health Choice Task Force meeting in December 1998.

Audiologists, pediatric dentists, pharmacists, and vision care providers were invited to participate with primary care providers because of new benefits available. This swift response helped shape and influence North Carolina's nationally recognized rollout of SCHIP in its early years of implementation. Concurrent with the outreach and enrollment efforts by state agencies, the Robert Wood Johnson Foundation made a $1 million supporting grant to one lead organization in each state under the auspices of a program called Covering Kids (CK). The NC Office of Rural Health (ORH) was the grant recipient, with Christine Kushner, MPA, as lead for ORH, and Sari Teplin, MS, MPH, as the program director. North Carolina's Covering Kids program engaged five counties (Buncombe, Cabarrus, Edgecombe, Forsyth, and Guilford) to evaluate outreach and enrollment strategies as a means of working out bottlenecks and administrative glitches in the procedures for getting children enrolled in either NC Health Choice or Medicaid.

In just two years, North Carolina reached a Health Choice enrollment of 69,678 children, just below the federal cap for the state. In January 2001, a state budget shortfall froze the immediate enrollment of children. Advocates adjusted by creating a waiting list of eligible children that reached more than 12,000 before the freeze was lifted. The pressure of a growing waiting list, publicized by media coverage and lobbying efforts, helped persuade the Governor and the General Assembly to find enough funds to reopen enrollment for a limited number of children on May 1, 2001. But the budgetary circumstances of a shortfall in tax revenue led to stops and restarts in appropriating state match for federal funds to maintain open enrollment for NC Health Choice. This circumstance would vex legislators, advocates, and families, plus all health providers who served NC Health Choice patients over consecutive years and multiple legislative sessions.

Despite the occasional chaos and faltering steps to create a health insurance program from scratch, NC Health Choice for Children was considered an unprecedented success for its fast rollout. Exceptional recognition is due to the problem-solving accomplished by the local county partners in the Covering Kids program, the quick engagement of the Health Choice Task Force by NCPeds, and members of numerous professional provider groups who came to the table. The outstanding performance of state employees leading work groups and directing the implementation of NC Health Choice made a real difference in the success of NC Health Choice. Some of these determined heroes include: June Milby and Barbara Brooks in the Division of Medical Assistance; Tom Vitaglione, Kevin Ryan, MD, Norma Marti, Carolyn Sexton, and Dianne Tyson in the Division of Public Health; Paul Sebo of the State Employees Health Plan, and Sandra Dodson of Blue Cross/Blue Shield of NC, the latter two agencies having the responsibility for managing the benefits implementation and fiscal operations of NC Health Choice. NCPeds Health Choice Task Force Chair Dr. Wally Brown would eventually turn over the leadership to Edward Davis, MD, FAAP, of Greenville, followed by Deborah Ainsworth, MD, FAAP, of Washington.

Simultaneously, a separate NC Health Choice Commission on Children with Special Health Care Needs was established from NC's special legislation to assure

> Despite the occasional chaos and faltering steps to create a health insurance program from scratch, NC Health Choice for Children was considered an unprecedented success for its fast rollout.

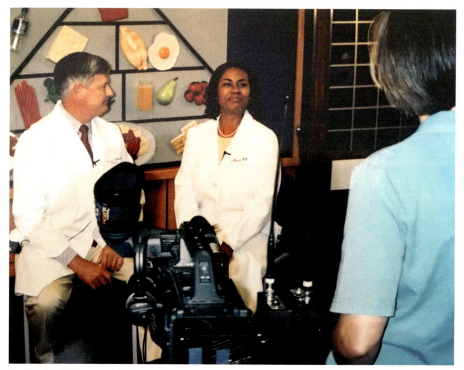

**Dr. Charles Willson and Dr. Laura Gerald record a TV PSA on obesity.**

that the children enrolled in Health Choice were receiving benefits comparable to those of Medicaid-eligible children. This group, co-chaired by Tom Vitaglione, MPH, and Dave Tayloe Jr., MD, FAAP, made sure that NCPeds recommendations for insurance coverage were implemented in Health Choice.

In 2001, The Robert Wood Johnson Foundation announced that the initial four-year grant program, Covering Kids, would end in 2002, but that a new round of funding would be forthcoming. The NC Office of Rural Health approached NCPeds about submitting the grant application to become the lead agency in North Carolina. The follow-up program was named Covering Kids and Families because some US states were now moving beyond SCHIP to expand Medicaid coverage for adults.

NCPeds successfully submitted the grant for $1 million to continue and expand the alliances for outreach and enrollment efforts achieved during the original grant. During the Chapter's grant-driven activities from 2003-2007, Patricia Garrett, PhD, was the program director, with Dr. Jane Foy serving as medical director. The Wake County Medical Society Foundation, led by Paul Harris, was a key ally in the grant application process, which required a 50 percent match from the grantee.

The Medical Society Foundation, with funding from the Raleigh-based John Rex Endowment, agreed to collaborate with NCPeds. Through this joint venture, NCPeds became North Carolina's lead agency for Covering Kids and Families and demonstrated the respected brand of the pediatric community as a dynamic influence for child health improvement.

Special funding from NCPeds was provided to Buncombe County Department of Social Services, Moore Health, a partnership between First Health of the Carolinas and the Moore County Chamber of Commerce, and the New Hanover County Partnership for Children (Smart Start). Events like putting flyers in Back-to-School packets for children to take home, and private and public partners providing information to employees of eligible children, including the University of North Carolina's sixteen campuses, the NC Hotel & Motel Association, and Aramark (a food and facilities management company), were organized. Adding public service announcements on local cable channels and major networks were strategies aimed at institutionalizing outreach and promoting the national toll-free number 1-877 KIDS NOW for enrollment assistance was accomplished by the NC Healthy Start Foundation led by Janice Freedman, MPH. The maneuvers, policy tweaks, and remarkable accomplishments, large and small, would fill a catalog and could not have happened without so many team members cooperating on a shared mission.

> NCPeds became North Carolina's lead agency for Covering Kids and Families and demonstrated the respected brand of the pediatric community as a dynamic influence for child health improvement.

Calls for enrollment assistance were routed to the NC Child Care Health and Safety Resource Center. The Resource Center hosted a switchboard for application assistance. North Carolina's Healthy Start Foundation printed applications in thirteen languages reflecting NC's expanding population and growing diversity. Jonathan Kotch, MD, FAAP, of the faculty at the UNC School of Public Health's Maternal and Child Health program, was the project director for the Resource Center. Jackie Quirk managed the call center, and interpreters handled live phone contact with families speaking English, Spanish, Creole, and French. Kotch's leadership on childcare safety and expanding the role of the Resource Center in assisting families to apply for NC Health Choice opened many doors to the childcare community comprised of hundreds of public and private businesses across the state. The NC Partnership for Children, better known as Smart Start, with a sponsored program in every one of North Carolina's one hundred counties, served as a catalyst through county Partnership boards and community contacts.

Besides printing all the Health Check and Health Choice materials, The Healthy Start Foundation served as a web host agency—an experimental but successful undertaking in the early 2000s—posting all the applications and outreach materials. Healthy Start also produced Public Service Announcements for television and radio, and complimented the efforts of the Covering Kids work groups by cooperating directly with state agencies to support outreach and enrollment.

The Robert Wood Johnson Foundation deserves commendation for launching Covering Kids and the second iteration, Covering Kids and Families, to enable the states to find and enroll eligible children in publicly funded health insurance. North Carolina's community of child health advocates in the public and private sectors identified in this commentary proved to be exceptional at putting the needs of children and families ahead of bureaucratic dominions.

## HEALTHY AND READY TO LEARN

The Children's Health Insurance Reauthorization Act (CHIPRA) in 2009 and the "Patient Protection and Affordable Care Act" in 2010 were signed by President Barack Obama. Numerous provisions in the law were celebrated for improving access to care for children, including no lifetime or annual limits to coverage, low or no copay for immunizations, coverage for preventive care, and allowing young adults up to age twenty-six to be covered through parents' insurance plans. These laws strengthened both Medicaid and the State Children's Health Insurance Program by extending reauthorization and appropriations.

The law also asserted consistent policy provisions that resolved and eliminated certain erratic and unresolved insurance regulations implemented among the predominantly federally funded but state-administered Medicaid and SCHIP programs. Both CHIPRA and the Affordable Care Act made funding available to the states for demonstrations to improve quality and to increase outreach and enrollment activities for families with children eligible for Medicaid or SCHIP. The law included the stipulation that one grant would be awarded per state. In North Carolina, Governor Beverly Perdue asked NCPeds to be the lead. The Governor's "Healthy and Ready to Learn" grant was awarded by the federal Department of Health and Human Services at the end of September, and immediately NCPeds started a search for a director and field staff to begin implementation.

At the January 2011 meeting of the State Coalition to Promote Health Insurance for Children, chaired by NCPeds, HRL Project Director Ania Boer, MPH, was introduced. Boer was a child health program veteran who had worked at the NC Healthy Start Foundation. Laura Brewer of Pembroke, Betty Macon of Roanoke Rapids, and India Foy of Greensboro were hired for field positions.

By March 2011, the HRL team had prepared the initial training events for school personnel in Davidson and Wayne counties to resume a strategically designed enrollment effort with funds for staffing to enroll eligible children for the first time since February 2007 when the Robert Wood Johnson Foundation's Covering Kids and Families project ended.

Healthy & Ready to Learn (HRL) was launched in sixteen North Carolina counties estimated to have high numbers of children eligible for government-subsidized insurance enrollment. Initial efforts were aimed at kindergartners who may be eligible but uninsured. The program was launched in cooperation with twenty-two local school systems (also called Local Education Authorities or LEAs). NCPeds negotiated a contract with each of the twenty-two local school systems to provide modest financial support for paper, printing, and staff to assist the HRL Coordinators in contacting teachers, counselors, and local child health advocates. Governor Perdue's office and State Superintendent of Public Instruction June Atkinson assisted NCPeds in working with school administrators, principals, nurses, and other personnel to give HRL high visibility and to help families enroll eligible children. NCPeds negotiated an agreement with the School Nurse Association of North Carolina as a key partner in designing and presenting the enrollment activities for each school system.

The state-mandated School Health Advisory Council (SHAC) in each local system supported the Healthy and Ready to Learn initiative which extended NCPeds influence with grass-roots leaders. The North Carolina Parent Teacher Association (NCPTA) was engaged as an active partner, communicating via its email membership numbering nearly 700,000 parents and teachers across the state.

HRL maintained an active presence on social media. Consistent with emerging innovations in the use of smartphones in the early 2010s, Healthy and Ready to Learn promoted a phone app developed by the NC Healthy Start Foundation with the name "NCfamilyhealth.org." By clicking on the app, capturing the QR scan code, or texting to a five-digit number, one could obtain accurate information on health insurance income eligibility status, how to initiate enrollment, and the types of health services available. This enabled outreach efforts to be distributed via social media methods popular with middle-school and high-school-age adolescents. Healthy and Ready to Learn continued operations through September 2013, when federal funding ended.

## HEALTH IMPROVEMENT INITIATIVES ON TOBACCO USE
## AND OBESITY REDUCTION 2002-2016

In July 2002, NCPeds agreed to take fiscal responsibility for the North Carolina Alliance for Health to manage all financial affairs for the Alliance, including the supervision of employees. This was done under the auspices of the 501(c)(3) status of the NCPeds Charitable Foundation.

The Alliance was created in 2002 as a formal but unincorporated coalition for the purpose of enacting statewide health improvement policies. Alliance funding came from "tobacco settlement" money that came to our state. The Alliance mission brought together many organizations under one umbrella to lobby the NC General Assembly to change statewide tobacco policy. Two goals were set: to increase the tax per pack on cigarettes, and to seek funding for associated strategies to reduce youth and adult smoking in North Carolina. This included a proposal to address second-hand smoke by creating a smoke-free workplace for all employees. Corporate and public institutions already started the movement to eliminate smoking in the workplace and on the campuses of government institutions.

The NC Health and Wellness Trust Fund Commission was already at work funding prevention with funding from the Tobacco Master Settlement Agreement with all US states concluded in 1998. During the Commission's tenure, three pediatricians served as Commissioners: Dr. Olson Huff of Asheville, Dr. Charles Willson of Farmville, and Dr. Jugta Kahai of Oak Island. A fourth pediatrician, Dr. Laura Gerald of Lumberton, served as the Commission's third executive director from 2010-2011. The Commission was abolished by a newly constituted legislature in 2011.

The Alliance built a large membership from its founding members in the early years, which included NCPeds, the American Heart Association, American Stroke Association, American Cancer Society Cancer Action Network, NC Prevention Partners, NC State Employees Association, NC Public Health Association, NC Association of Local Health Directors, and NC Academy of Family Physicians. Eventually, several dozen health advocacy organizations, including the NC Conservation Council, Christian Action League, NC Council of Churches, Covenant with NC's Children, Healthy Carolinians, First Health of the Carolinas, Be Active NC, HOPSports, Active Living by Design, NC School Nutrition Association, NC Association of Athletic, Physical Education, Recreation and Dance Instructors and Teachers, NC Eat Smart and Move More, UNC School of Public Health Alumni Association, and American Diabetes Association became participating members. National partners included the Americans for Non-Smokers' Rights Foundation, and The Campaign for Tobacco-Free Kids.

The Alliance broadened its appeal to North Carolina's African American and Latinx populations and welcomed the influential organizations The Old North State

Medical Society and El Pueblo. The Alliance also welcomed several dozen individual members representing numerous other organizations that supported the agenda.

The Alliance savored a victory benefitting children during the 2003 legislative session. State Senator Bill Purcell, MD, FAAP, a pediatrician representing Scotland County, filed a bill titled "Tobacco Free Schools," requiring local school boards to develop written policies prohibiting the use of tobacco products in public school buildings. The bill passed and was ratified to become law. The North Carolina legislature's traditional automatic rejection of any legislation designed to reduce smoking and affect tobacco's "sacred" economic power in the

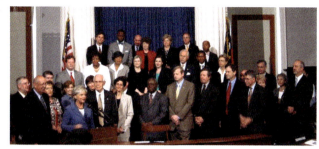

**Governor Bev Perdue signs legislation for smoke-free restaurants. NCPeds' Dr. William Purcell, cochair of the Senate Health Committee, was a leader in achieving the victory.**

state now appeared vulnerable to new evidence-based arguments.

A key advisor and consultant to the membership and leadership team of the Alliance was the NC Division of Public Health's Tobacco Prevention and Control Branch, led by Sally Herndon, MPH. While state agencies were prohibited from membership or lobbying activities, this affiliation was important to inform policy initiatives and to gain a perspective on existing state assets and resources that matched the Alliance's mission and objectives. During the lobbying effort to pass the bill, the Alliance secured funding from the Campaign for Tobacco-Free Kids program and created a public service announcement in support of the bill that featured former University of North Carolina basketball coach Dean Smith.

The Alliance achieved a major goal when North Carolina enacted the first increase in the tax on cigarettes and tobacco products since 1993 by increasing the rate from $.05 per pack (50th among states at the time) to $.30 per pack in 2005, a six-fold increase, with another $.05 per pack added in 2006 for a total of $.35 per pack. The Alliance had proposed a $.75 per pack increase, but NC's strong tobacco lobby, including multiple legacy tobacco companies located in North Carolina and rural legislators representing tobacco farmers—still a significant agricultural and economic engine for the state at this time—successfully negotiated a reduction. The NC Alliance for Health members, including pediatricians from NCPeds, constituted a powerful voice to raise the tax since tobacco tax increases have been proven to reduce youth smoking.

The Alliance agenda expanded in 2005 to address the widely recognized obesity crisis among children and adults. Bob Schwartz, MD, FAAP, was instrumental in helping launch Eat Smart Move More North Carolina in 2002. Supported by the NC Division of Public Health, Eat Smart Move More NC invited business, community, faith, public health, medical school, and university representatives to create a statewide initiative to address healthy eating, active lifestyles, and achieving a healthy weight. Eat Smart Move More NC soon became an active and cooperating member of the Alliance.

In the legislature, the Alliance addressed the need to eliminate sugar-sweetened beverages and processed snack foods from the vending machines in public schools, promoted healthy physical education policies and practices for kindergarten through eighth-grade students, advocated for nutrition standards to improve healthy eating, and supported optimal pricing for child nutrition program food and supplies. In later years, the Alliance promoted initiatives supporting local, sustainable food producers, and policy changes to allow eligible recipients to use Food Stamps and SNAP benefits to purchase healthy foods at farmers' markets. The legislature enacted a number of provisions in response to the Alliance's educational efforts and leadership in collaboration with local school advocates, Eat Smart Move More NC, The State Board of Education, and the NC Department of Public Instruction.

In 2008, the Alliance's goal of enacting legislation to create smoke-free workplaces statewide was narrowly defeated in the legislative session. In 2009, following a Presidential election year, the Alliance went back to work. Under the shrewd leadership of Dr. Purcell, Co-Chair of the Senate Health Committee, and the House Majority Leader, Representative Hugh Holliman of Davidson County, a lung cancer survivor, the Alliance realized its goal. In May 2009, the General Assembly passed compromise legislation to create a smoke-free environment in all restaurants and bars across North Carolina, effective January 2, 2010.

The implementation of smoke-free bars and restaurants immediately improved the health of North Carolinians, as comparative studies of air quality showed that emergency department visits for heart and asthma attacks decreased by 21 percent in the first year. With public acceptance polling at 83 percent approval and with compliance being nearly universal, this constituted a policy "home run." The Alliance was instrumental in educating legislators about environmental science and public health studies demonstrating the advantages of an indoor smoke-free policy. In the aftermath of implementation, a legal challenge to the smoke-free law was defeated before the NC Supreme Court.

# Improving Quality, Efficiency, and Payment in Pediatric Practice

**by Graham Barden, III, MD, FAAP; Christoph Diasio, MD, FAAP**

I have long had an interest in pediatric practice management as a tool to make private community-based pediatrics a viable healthcare delivery system. My father started our practice in 1952. Although he was quite good as a pediatrician, he had no interest in practice management. When I joined my father's group in 1985, it was clear that I could contribute by learning as much as I could about practice management.

I went to my first NC Pediatric Society (NCPeds) meeting in Asheville at the Grove Park Inn in the 1980s, and saw NCPeds give a slew of awards to state employees for doing wonderful things. All the docs applauded them, and they were beaming from the recognition. I thought, "That's genius and I want in!" It was obvious that there are people all over the state in lots of non-medical jobs trying just as hard as pediatricians to improve children's health and outcomes. I was hooked—and wanted in.

I met Joe Ponzi, a pediatrician in Goldsboro, at the meeting, and he became my mentor, teaching me about managing a practice. I met Bill Hubbard, NCPeds president from 2000–02, who shared an interest in computers and invited me in 2002 to participate in an interest group centered around computers and management. I continued going to the annual meetings to learn about pediatrics and management. In 2006, NCPeds President Herb Clegg called Christoph Diasio, a young pediatrician in Southern Pines, and me to see if we could start a pediatric council to more formally help pediatricians around the state to operate more efficient practices in a rapidly changing world.

The American Academy of Pediatrics had begun to encourage state chapters to create pediatric councils to assist pediatricians with practice management. We agreed and it has been a wonderful learning experience with lots of late nights getting into the weeds of the business of pediatrics. We were charged with trying to keep private practices financially viable, whether that meant convincing insurance companies to pay better, or to help practices solve the same back-office issues we all have.

Having an official name—NC Pediatric Council—allowed us to operate on behalf of all our members and opened doors for us to meet with state government and private insurance company officials with whom an individual practicing pediatrician might not have enough standing to do. Yet those officials needed to hear from front-line pediatricians.

In 1994, NC's Immunization Branch implemented the federal Vaccines for Children (VFC) program and the NC Universal Childhood Distribution Program

Having an official name—NC Pediatric Council— allowed us to operate on behalf of all our members and opened doors for us to meet with state government and private insurance company officials with whom an individual practicing pediatrician might not have enough standing to do.

simultaneously. This allowed practicing pediatricians to receive free vaccines paid for by a combination of state and federal dollars, and to be paid a state-approved vaccine administration fee for giving vaccines to all children in their practices. Before 1994, vaccine costs had to be covered by revenues collected for well-child visits; Medicaid and private insurance companies did not reimburse pediatricians for their vaccine product or vaccine administration costs.

The state approved an administration payment for public and private payers of $13.71 for the first injection—the highest recommended administration fee for the state under VFC guidelines. The payment for two or more injections was set at $25.00, because the NC Commission on Health Services did not think parents would pay more than that amount for administration of all vaccines needed at a given visit, and if the patients left the physicians' offices unvaccinated, their caretakers were unlikely to follow through by taking them to a health department for vaccines provided by the state. There was no administration payment for the oral polio vaccine (OPV).

In 1994, excluding flu, there were only seventeen vaccinations during childhood, and no visit required more than two shots. By 2006, it was clear that vaccinations had become central to pediatric practice. That year there were thirty-one vaccinations required (excluding flu), with only nineteen of the thirty-one earning the $13.71. The average payment for administration had fallen to $8.40, when taking into consideration that physicians would only receive $25.00 if giving any number of vaccines at a given office visit. Nationally, there was a great focus on covering the cost of vaccination through the administration fees. To help the cause, the AAP developed The Business Case for Pricing Vaccines and Immunization Administration. Vaccine product cost and administration fees took center stage for pediatric councils.

The NC Pediatric Council started with its first conference call in 2006. We were concerned about the following:

1. Blue Cross Blue Shield of North Carolina (BCBSNC) would not pay for administration of vaccines beyond two, even if using privately purchased (not government-funded) vaccines;

2. BCBS State Employees' Health Plan (SEHP) would not pay for more than two administration fees;

3. Medicaid had not yet started to pay for more than two vaccine administrations, which Steve Wegner, MD, FAAP, of Community Care of NC (Medicaid) and Dave Tayloe Jr., MD, pediatrician in private practice in Goldsboro, had convinced them to do;

4. Caps apply only to VFC eligible children;

5. Lobbying Medicaid to allow practices to distribute asthma durable medical equipment (DME) (nebulizer machines, masks and tubing for nebulizer machines, spacers) without needing to become a DME provider; and,

6. Improving communication among our members by regularly contacting a directory of key people, and to create a listserv for better communication.

Because of the tremendous flood of new vaccinations, we supported moving to a two-tier program with VFC vaccine for uninsured/under-insured and Medicaid-eligible children and private vaccines for all others. Although a bit more complicated to coordinate storage and record-keeping for state and private vaccines, it allowed pediatricians to make some margin on both the vaccine product and the vaccine administration service.

To help keep private practice viable, we now focused on making vaccination the cornerstone of a healthy pediatric practice. NCPeds always has had exceptionally good representation on AAP national committees. In 2011, the chapter nominated me, and I was appointed to a position on the COPAM (Committee on Practice and Ambulatory Medicine) that was designed to be the AAP coordinating council for all vaccine issues.

The following year, a report was released from the Office of the Inspector General showing that the nation's physicians were not doing well with the technical aspects of VFC vaccine storage. For the next several years, Christoph and I studied, experimented with, and promoted better storage methods for office practices in partnership with the NC Immunization Branch.

In May 2013, we went with two AAP staff members and AAP Board Member Sara Goza (who was the subsequent AAP president) to the Centers for Disease Control (CDC) in Atlanta to meet with Dr. Chesley Richards, director of their Immunization Services Division, National Center for Immunization and Respiratory Diseases (NCIRD). Our goal was to see if we could partner with the CDC to promote better vaccine storage practices by physicians. We wanted to focus on better equipment, use of phone-aware thermometers, education, and fewer paperwork documentation requirements.

I gave a presentation for the biannual NC Immunization Branch conference on the mechanics of vaccine storage, published an article in AAP News on vaccine transport, created an AAP Storage and Handling course, and wrote disaster planning and recovery articles. I was unable to effect much change within the CDC, so I went to Washington, DC, to meet at National Institute of Standards and Technology (NIST) with Michal Chojnacky, who did the testing for the CDC vaccine storage program. She was thrilled to have a practicing pediatrician interested in her work, and she subsequently promoted my use of conditioned frozen water bottles for emergency transport of vaccines.

## NC TRACKS AND NCPEDS PRACTICE MANAGERS' LISTSERV

Steve Shore invited the Pediatric Council (Christoph Diasio and me) to participate in a monthly multidisciplinary state group beginning January 2014. We were tasked with helping the state implement the newly passed Affordable Care Act (ACA) and the state's new comprehensive computer system, NC Tracks. That tradition,

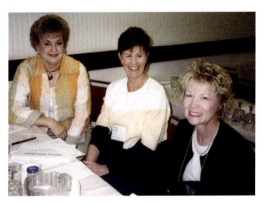

Left to Right: Carol Jarvis (Thomasville), Nancy Coggins (Raleigh), and Debbie Cashion (Hickory) at the annual Practice Managers Retreat

which continues now, has served NCPeds well in avoiding an adversarial relationship between pediatricians and the state. Both sides have learned to trust the other in their joint efforts to solve practice problems and improve child health.

NC Tracks was the new comprehensive computer system designed to handle all payments for NC Medicaid. It was the first new system since 1978, and it was a pretty rough start, especially with the ACA starting at the same time. But the best invention of the Pediatric Council, and the most valuable to date for support of private pediatric practice, was the creation of the practice managers' listserv, already an effective communications tool organized by NCPeds in 2003. All member practices were invited to sign up their practice administrators for the email list and to encourage them to participate in Practice Managers' Section meetings at the annual meeting.

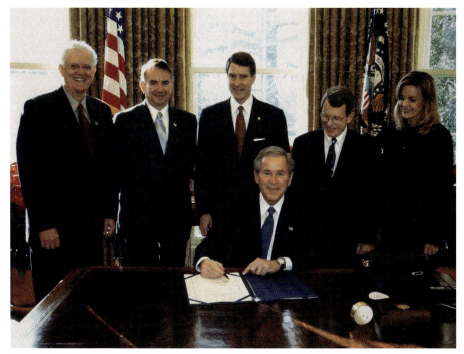

Standing behind President George Bush, left to right: Steve Edwards, representing AAP; Tommy Thompson, Secretary of Health and Human Services; Bill Frist, Senate Majority Leader; Senator Mike DeWine (current governor of Ohio), who introduced the Bill that became the Best Pharmaceuticals for Children Act; and a pharmaceutical representative.

During the implementation of the ACA and NC Tracks, misinformation and no information were the major barriers to efficient participation by practices. We promoted and supported practice managers from all over the state to ask questions and to compete for discovering the best solution to each other's questions and problems. This network continues to strengthen our private practices across the state.

### AFFORDABLE CARE ACT (ACA)

We dove into the weeds of the ACA to make sure we took advantage of every possible advantage available to physicians. Christoph noticed the first problem; NC Tracks was programmed using the 2013 multiplier for Medicaid payment, rather than the more favorable 2009 multiplier. That one change boosted payments for the state's primary care physicians by three percent. In addition, the state was not planning on paying ACA rates for anything but sick Evaluation and Management (E&M) codes. The Well-Child Codes (WCC) had an "EP" modifier, which stands for EPSDT: Early Periodic Screening Diagnosis and Treatment, the traditional terminology for well-child encounters in Medicaid. Because the administration codes had a different modifier, the Division of Medical Assistance (DMA) insisted that the presence of modifiers disqualified those codes from ACA payment enhancements! DMA was trying to be extremely careful to follow exactly what the ACA seemed to be mandating. We felt strongly that the purpose of the ACA was to give more financial support to primary care physicians, and that meant the ACA enhancement should be applied to all well-child codes and vaccine administration codes. But to have ACA applied to WCC codes, the codes had to be unbundled, since a Medicaid well visit included much more than just the services included in E&M. For DMA administrators, unbundling was incomprehensible. We proposed a cleaner, more accurate method that increased the ACA payment by an average of twelve dollars per visit—a substantial improvement. DMA eventually accepted our proposal.

These changes were happening at the same time as the implementation of NC Tracks. There were many glitches in the sign-up procedures, and many physicians were going to miss the attestation requirement. NC Pediatric Council lobbied hard, and was able to extend the attestation period by a full year—from June 30, 2013, to June 30, 2014. This increased the number of attested primary care physicians from 5,000 to 16,000! Plus, the council convinced the state to make all claims submitted for services rendered between January 1, 2013, and December 31, 2014, regardless of date of submission, payable retroactively to January 2013 for the two-year "bump" period designated by the ACA.

## ADDITIONAL ACCOMPLISHMENTS

The NCPeds Pediatric Council convinced the state that the vaccine administration fee for the ACA was to be paid at $20.45, even if the practice had billed only $13.71, as previously required by the NC Immunization Branch, for the two-year "bump" period designated by the ACA. Better yet, the enhanced payment would be pushed out to the practices with the higher amount, without having to refile old claims! Physicians were allowed to re-submit the claims if they had not used the ACA-allowed increase for 2013-14. The council also convinced the state to eliminate the five dollar copay for NC Health Choice or CHIP (Child Health Insurance Program) well-child services.

We were able to circumvent the poor service from the NC Tracks Help Desk—they were totally overwhelmed during the switch-over—by using our NCPeds Practice Managers' Listserv to detect problems and to crowd-source solutions, then convince the state to implement solutions to common problems.

The new 2014 National Correct Coding Initiative (NCCI) edits were inappropriately applied to Day of Services (DOS) 2013 visits, which resulted in many denied claims. We established that 2014 rules could not be applied to 2013 visits. The new $20.45 ACA administration payments did not begin for 2013 visits until

May 2014. There were a lot of missteps that had to be resolved, and eventually were approved in our favor.

We realized for the ACA, there was only one payment value available for all vaccine administration codes, and that value was $20.45. It was wrong for the state to have paid a reduced amount, $11.00, for subsequent vaccinations (90472 or 90474) at a single visit. During our first Wednesday conference call in January 2015, we obtained a commitment for the state to sweep all payments for vaccine administration back to January 1, 2013, and pay at the higher $20.45 rate. The reprocessing was to happen in March 2015, but once again, it did not happen on schedule.

By April 2016, DMA said the state would not pay the single $20.45 going back to January 1, 2013, and could not renegotiate with the federal Centers for Medicare and Medicaid Services (CMS) unless it was mispaid. We contacted several of the large practices in the state and explained to the leaders that we had a particularly good case for better, and fair payment, which could be won in court. We asked that they file the tort claim in their name—not NCPeds—and all initially chip in $5,000 with a commitment for another $5,000, if needed.

For a ten-provider practice with 40 percent Medicaid patient population, the upside was at least $200,000 per practice if we won. We convinced eight practices to contribute, as well as lesser amounts from smaller practices. We hired Joey Ponzi, JD, a lawyer who was the son of Dr. Joe Ponzi, MD, of Goldsboro Pediatrics. The NC Pediatric Society was a friend of the suit, as was the NC Academy of Family Physicians. We eventually won the lawsuit to pay a single higher administration fee based on the wording of the ACA and the State Plan Amendment (SPA). This compelled CMS and the state to pay the differential of approximately $18 million dollars to all ACA primary care physicians in the state. Total legal fees were $80,000, paid primarily by the initial large groups, but complemented by contributions from many other practices in the state. There was no cost to NCPeds. In fact, the society reaped a substantial "war chest" of donations from thankful members who understood that it might be necessary for the chapter to do this again if the need arises! The largest single contributor by way of discounted fees was our lawyer, Joey Ponzi. We appreciated the "family discount!"

On reflection, the most interesting part of the suit was that it was handled as a business dispute among friends. The state could not pay us unless we successfully sued the state. There was no animosity on either side, and we have continued to have the monthly "First Wednesday" meetings that began in 2014. We just do not talk about the suit during those sessions. I believe, if anything, this experience strengthened our relationship with the Department of Health and Human Services, and strengthened the foundation we would need to successfully navigate Medicaid Transformation in 2021. Truly remarkable!

For me, the "Secret Sauce" of NCPeds has been the incredible donation of time and enthusiasm given freely by our members. What got us fired up to participate was the tradition that any member could join the executive committee meetings if they just arrived at the annual and quarterly meetings a few hours early and paid their own way in terms of travel and lodging. That also allows the most interested members to "bubble up," and become part of the leadership and move forward to become officers. It is infectious to see the amount of effort that goes on behind the scenes.

# Redesigning Foster Care

by Marian Earls, MD, MTS, FAAP

NCPeds has an established history of supporting innovation and quality improvement in pediatric health care. An example of this is the pediatric leadership that has led to the Fostering Health NC Program.

By 2008, we had had many conversations in the NCPeds Mental Health Committee about children and youth in foster care. As I started my NCPeds presidency for the years 2008–10, I authored a white paper on the need for continuity, socio-emotional support, and systems coordination for children and youth in foster care. We shared this with The Duke Endowment and were given a year's planning grant to develop a project jointly with the South Carolina Chapter.

We worked for that year on optimal processes and standards for care. With the economic downturn, however, The Duke Endowment did not renew funding for implementation. I came to Community Care of NC (CCNC), the physician-directed management entity for the NC Medicaid Program, as director of pediatric programs in 2010—at first part-time, then full-time in 2012. North Carolina was one of ten applicants of the eighteen states that applied to receive the Child Health Insurance Program Reauthorization Act (CHIPRA) Quality Demonstration Grant in 2010. I led the CHIPRA Grant from 2010-15, and our team identified early that foster care would be an area of focus.

Through this large grant, we were able to fund NCPeds to hire staff to lead a state advisory group of important stakeholders, including: Department of Social Services (DSS); local and state public health agencies; pediatricians already leading clinics for children in foster care; foster parents; private foster care agencies; Strong Able Youth Speaking Out (SAYSO)—an organization for youth who had transitioned out of foster care between the ages of fourteen and twenty-four; Care Coordination for Children (CC4C), now called Care Management for At Risk Children (CMARC)—the birth to age five Medicaid care coordination program based in local health departments; CCNC Care Management; CCNC pharmacists; and CCNC data analysts.

The work group outlined the core elements for a collaborative system among pediatric practices—CMARC, CCNC Care Managers, and the Department of Social Services (DSS) at the local level. NCPeds' foster care staff began recruiting county DSSs, local pediatric practices, and CCNC Networks to commit to: implementing the core elements of the AAP Healthy Foster Care America guidelines; involvement of CC4C for all children under age five; CCNC Care Managers for those older than age five; and agreements for communication and continuity of records. The work continues, and currently most county DSS agencies participate in Fostering Health NC. Subsequent to the CHIPRA funding, NCPeds now has a contract with DSS at the state level Division of Social Services to implement Fostering Health NC (FHNC). Fostering Health NC has received an award from the National Center for Medical Home.

The cross-sector collaboration led by Fostering Health NC has resulted in a collection of products for assuring medical homes for children and youth in foster care; continuity of records; review of medications; routine social-emotional assessment in the medical home; enhanced schedule of follow-up visits; standardized initial and comprehensive visits in collaboration with the DSS worker; and best practice principles for transition of youth out of foster care. Guidelines and tools for primary care clinicians, care managers, DSS workers, and foster parents are on the NCPeds Fostering Health NC website (www.ncpeds.org).

> Fostering Health NC has received an award from the National Center for Medical Home.

Under the Fostering Health NC protocols, foster children have an office visit with a primary care provider within one week of placement; a complete physical (EPSDT: Early Periodic Screening Diagnosis and Treatment) within one month; and then office visits every three to six months going forward. Primary care physicians have learned to link all foster children with mental health professionals.

NCPeds Fostering Health NC continues to convene the state advisory group, as well as the Transition Age Youth and Former Foster Youth work group, Medication work group, and Private Agency work group. In addition, NCPeds staff operate a robust website sharing multiple resources. FHNC has assisted DSS with the state's Health Care Oversight and Coordination Plan (HOCP), pharmacology monitoring, and data for improvement needs.

# Medical Liability and Children

**by John Rusher, JD, MD, FAAP**

NCPeds has always been active in proposing and supporting legislation that protects children and pediatricians. To do that effectively, NCPeds has stayed attuned to the political atmosphere in the General Assembly, collaborating with allies such as the North Carolina Medical Society, NC Medical Mutual Insurance Company (now named Curi), the main medical liability company in our state, and effective lobbyists.

As an example, in 2011, there was a significant shift in the North Carolina General Assembly to a Republican majority in both Houses. The new leadership listed medical liability reform as one of its top priorities, and in February 2011, a malpractice and tort reform bill was introduced. A six-month battle ensued between the trial attorneys' organization, known as Advocates for Justice, and the North Carolina Medical Society.

In July 2011, the bill was finally enacted into law by an override of the governor's veto. The key provisions in the bill that the North Carolina Medical Society had pushed included a cap on noneconomic damages of $500,000, the establishment of appeal bonds for large jury awards, and the requirement that claims made on behalf of minors be brought in a more timely manner.

NCPeds worked closely with the North Carolina Medical Society in supporting the tort reform bill. In addition, the advocacy of NCPeds was instrumental in effecting the change in the statute of limitations for alleged malpractice affecting children because this was an issue that impacted pediatricians the most.

Before 2011, a child who alleged harm by a physician or other medical worker could bring a malpractice action within three years of the injury (four years if the injury is not reasonably discovered within the first two years) or before turning nineteen, whichever was later. The statute of limitations was the same regardless of whether the child alleging harm was younger than ten or younger than eighteen at the time of the alleged harm. As a result, physicians faced potential claims arising from the care provided to a young child for nearly two decades after the provided care.

A landmark vaccine liability case in our state involved a vaccine given in 1974 that went to a jury trial in 1985. By 1985, no one knew which vaccine manufacturer made the vaccine in question in the 1974 event, so the pediatricians became the "deep pockets" in the medical malpractice lawsuit (see *Big Dave: Visionary Leader*).

The revised statute provides that if a child is younger than ten when the alleged harm occurs, the medical malpractice claim must be brought within three years of the injury or before turning ten, whichever is later. If the child is older than ten when

The advocacy of NCPeds was instrumental in effecting the change in the statute of limitations for alleged malpractice affecting children because this was an issue that impacted pediatricians the most.

the alleged malpractice occurs, the statute remains at the previous level—the suit must be brought within three years of the injury or before the child turns nineteen, whichever is later.

The tort reform bill enacted by the General Assembly, including the changes to the statute of limitations pushed by NCPeds, significantly reduced malpractice cases against physicians.

## State-Funded 24-Hour Hotline for Breastfeeding Mothers

**by Emily Hannon, MD, IBCLC, FAAP**

When I was growing up, my dad always taught me the value of networking. I remember rolling my eyes as a teenager and thinking that networking was just something for people who did not want to put in the time or energy to get ahead. It was a lot easier to just talk to people at a cocktail party about what you wanted and assume they could connect you with the right people. I thought it was much harder and ultimately more rewarding to do the hard work myself and not take help from "connected" people. Clearly, my teenaged brain did not realize the true value of networking in a tight-knit professional community like the pediatric community in North Carolina.

I spent the first ten years of my career as a practicing pediatrician in California, the most populous state in the country. While I loved the group I practiced with, I felt disconnected from the statewide pediatric community. There were four state chapters of the AAP, making it difficult to really get to know other pediatricians. Four years ago, my family and I moved across the country to North Carolina for my husband's job. We had no connection to the area, so I knew no one, let alone pediatricians.

About two months after arriving, I attended the North Carolina Pediatric Society (NCPeds) Winter Open Forum. I did not know what to expect, but because I was in the midst of a job hunt, I thought it would be good to meet some pediatricians. What I experienced was very different from what I had experienced during other state AAP meetings. Since the meeting did not occur during the annual meeting, it was smaller by definition. In a room of about fifty other pediatricians, we passed around a microphone to introduce ourselves. People cheered when I said I had just arrived two months earlier. That day I met the current NCPeds president and a former NCPeds president who had also served as the national AAP president. I spent the day learning with my new state colleagues.

Being in a smaller state has allowed me to get involved on a statewide level in a way that I had not been able to be involved in before. Shortly after arriving, I asked if anyone needed help with breastfeeding support and education (my area of specialization). The NCPeds executive director introduced me to the AAP chapter breastfeeding coordinator for North Carolina. When I asked if I could help her, she said, "Sure! Let's be co-coordinators!" Her welcoming attitude allowed me to jump right in and be involved.

As an AAP chapter breastfeeding coordinator (CBC), I have been able to meet other states' CBCs. During one meeting, the CBC from Ohio mentioned that she helped start a twenty-four-hour statewide breastfeeding hotline, a resource that families in her state could use to obtain free breastfeeding support any time of day or night. I wanted to know more and explore starting a similar service in North Carolina, so I reached out to her, and she became my project mentor.

I had been thinking about the idea of a statewide breastfeeding hotline for a while when I attended a pediatric grand rounds at a nearby academic medical center. The speaker was a former NCPeds president and past AAP president—the same one I had met two years earlier at the small winter open forum when I was brand new to the state. He spoke of advocacy and how a community pediatrician in a small North Carolina town could affect change on a statewide and national level through connections— what he called "networking." At the end of his talk, he offered audience members his assistance with advocacy projects they had been considering. He said we could call or email him anytime.

I waited about an hour to email him. (I did not want to seem too eager!) I told him my idea to replicate the successful statewide breastfeeding hotline in North Carolina. He listened, then carefully outlined the dozens of people with whom I should talk. He introduced me to many people via email, setting the stage for my continued planning. Through that initial introductory email after grand rounds, I have collaborated with and gleaned ideas from many key players in our state: section chiefs in the Department of Health and Human Services Division of Public Health; leaders of statewide breastfeeding coalitions; heads of grassroots maternal advocacy organizations; leaders of the North Carolina Institute of Medicine, Child Fatality

Task Force, and Medicaid. My NC colleagues even connected me with key people in a neighboring southern state that had data showing the cost and benefits of running a successful breastfeeding hotline program. I now know these people by name. They know me by name, and more importantly, they are invested in the statewide breastfeeding hotline project. Every one of them has, at some point, said, "I like this idea. You know who you should talk to is . . ." Then I connect with that person, and the domino chain keeps going. While it is still a work in progress, the more people I meet and tell about the idea, the more support I receive, which makes me very hopeful.

I had no idea that moving to North Carolina would provide me with an opportunity to be involved so directly in an effort to improve the health, well-being, and support for families on a statewide level. The connections I have made through my "networking" have allowed me to move my project forward, have made me feel connected with my pediatric colleagues, and would make my dad proud.

In the NC Department of Health and Human Services 2023-24 State Action Plan for Nutrition Security, the statewide breastfeeding hotline has been adopted as one of two initiatives to increase breastfeeding support and rates by submitting a Medicaid State Plan Amendment. The second initiative includes breastfeeding training for women, infants, and children's (WIC) personnel.

## An Advocacy Journey: Paid Family and Medical Leave (PFML)

by Kimberly Montez, MD, MPH, FAAP

Given my own experience with the lack of parental leave following the premature birth of my daughter, I became passionate about advocating for paid family and medical leave policies. Working at a federally qualified community health center when I had my daughter, I also realized that many low-income patients and families, particularly those of color, were disproportionately impacted by not having access to paid leave. In my mind, the passage of a national paid leave program is essential for promoting health equity, given the racial and ethnic disparities in infant outcomes.

My passion turned into action when I attended an NCPeds Winter Open Forum with a speakers' panel of leaders of advocacy organizations, including MomsRising. During the panel, the organizations laid out their advocacy agendas, which included PFML, and encouraged partnerships with pediatricians to promote family-friendly policies. Recognizing the power of my voice as a mom and pediatrician, I was excited to embark on an advocacy journey with the support of NCPeds and MomsRising. Elizabeth Hudgins, NCPeds executive director, facilitated my connection with

MomsRising, whose team helped me publish an opinion-editorial (op-ed) in my local newspaper.

This media advocacy opened the door for additional advocacy efforts, including national opportunities. A producer from National Public Radio's (NPR) On Point found my online op-ed and invited me to a radio show along with Katy Tur, an MSNBC news anchor, who had just devoted a segment on her show to PFML. Following my appearance on NPR, Katy Tur's team reached out to interview me for an NBC Nightly News segment, during which Katy Tur followed Alex Ohanian (husband to Serena Williams and Reddit co-founder). Mr. Ohanian promoted paid leave for the US (PL+US campaign), and he advocates for "dadvocates" on Capitol Hill to advocate for PFML. PL+US later featured me in a report about employer trends in PFML policies. After appearing on NPR's On Point, an NPR producer for Charlotte Talks invited me to a show about PFML, during which I was connected with New America's Vicki Shabo, an expert in PFML policies. I later reached out to Vicki Shabo to collaborate on a perspectives piece on PFML as a health equity policy published in *PEDIATRICS*.

> As a very active member of NCPeds, I will always enthusiastically share how this group has engaged me personally on my advocacy journey for the children and families of our state and nation. Children's lives depend on it!

Given the recent momentum around paid leave, North Carolina's partnership with MomsRising has continued, and we have collaborated on several advocacy opportunities related to PFML in NC. These efforts have included being an invited keynote speaker at the Think Babies™ Strolling Thunder Rally and presenting at the Injury-Free NC Academy about the "Disparities in Family-Friendly Workplace Policies" for injury and violence prevention practitioners. MomsRising again collaborated with me on an op-ed urging NC legislators to enact PFML, published in the *Charlotte Observer* and the *News & Observer* (Raleigh), and we have submitted a commentary on the importance of family-friendly policies to the *North Carolina Medical Journal*.

From a legislative advocacy standpoint, I have advocated for PFML in person and through countless emails and calls with many of my representatives at the NC General Assembly in Raleigh. Additionally, along with MomsRising, I was an invited speaker at the North Carolina Child Fatality Task Force, a legislative study commission that makes recommendations to the General Assembly about how to reduce child deaths. When NC legislators introduced paid leave bills this year, I was an invited speaker at the press conference. With the assistance of MomsRising, a group of advocates met virtually with US House Rep. Kathy E. Manning's staff to discuss PFML; Rep. Manning represents NC Congressional District Six. Although NC is not yet among the twelve states plus Puerto Rico and Washington, DC, with paid leave policies, I will continue to advocate for passage of PFML in NC through media and legislative advocacy.

In order to amplify the voice of pediatricians in the national conversation around PFML, I collaborated with the AAP Section on Perinatal Medicine (SOPM) as a lead author on a 2020 AAP Annual Leadership Forum (ALF) resolution on the importance of advocacy for PFML, which reached number eight within the top ten resolutions ranked by ALF attendees. In conjunction with the SOPM, the section on breastfeeding, and the Council on Community Pediatrics, I am the lead author on a new AAP policy statement and an accompanying technical report on PFML, which were approved for fast-track status by the AAP Board of Directors. Lastly, I was an invited speaker for two educational sessions at the 2021 AAP National Conference and Exhibition to educate and inspire other pediatricians about the importance of PFML advocacy as an opportunity to promote health equity among their patients.

Although I never imagined where my advocacy journey would lead me, it all started with the encouragement and support of NCPeds and a winter open forum. NCPeds made it possible for me to collaborate with partners through social media, scholarly publications, and policy advocacy; regularly engage with legislators through meetings, letters, and phone calls; educate trainees and other child health professionals; and partner with the national AAP. I endeavor to improve child health and mitigate disparities by persistently advocating for the passage of a comprehensive national paid family and medical leave program, which is just within reach. As a very active member of NCPeds, I will always enthusiastically share how this group has engaged me personally on my advocacy journey for the children and families of our state and nation. Children's lives depend on it!

# The Value of Pediatrician Advocates for Transgender Youth

by Emily Vander Schaff, MD, MPH, FAAP

Transgender children, like all children, want to belong. In 2021, when their health and well-being were threatened, North Carolina pediatricians stood up quickly and effectively in their support.

In 2020, the United States experienced a flurry of strikingly similar legislative efforts aimed at limiting the rights of transgender youth in states across the nation. One type of legislation sought to restrict children to play only on sports teams aligned with their assigned sex at birth. Another sought to prohibit clinicians from providing gender-affirming clinical care to adolescents and young adults. Pediatricians in North Carolina knew the harm that the passage of these bills could cause for children in the state. They acted quickly.

Bills restricting high school athletes to teams aligning with assigned sex at birth threatened to undermine many transgender (and intersex) youths' ability to build community and self-esteem. These policies are difficult and invasive to enforce. In many states, including North Carolina, they are made unnecessary by existing athletics rules offering clear guidance around team participation by lived-in gender identity.[5] Bills prohibiting clinicians from prescribing puberty-pausing and hormonal medications to transgender children and young adults would have forced children to undergo unwanted and irreversible changes to their bodies, leading to great preventable psychological distress. Importantly, such bills also disrupt the clinician-patient relationship, creating a dangerous precedent of elected public officials determining the "standard of medical care" in the absence of guidance from the medical profession.

Both bills sent powerful, direct, and harmful messages to children already at high risk of psychological distress. More than one-half of transgender youth have considered suicide and one-third have attempted it. The risk of suicide rises with bullying, exclusion, rejection, and lack of social and societal support and affirmation.[6] Conversely, children whose gender identity is affirmed are at reduced risk of suicide.[7] Pediatricians considered it especially destructive and dangerous that these bills were introduced all across the country during a global pandemic when at least a quarter of all children and adolescents were experiencing depression[8] and when they longed for community the most.

---

[5] North Carolina High School Athletic Association Student Requirements for Interscholastic Athletic Participation. Last accessed March 24, 2021: https://www.nchsaa.org/sites/default/files/attachments/Section%201.pdf

[6] Olson , Kristina R. PhD, Lily Durwood BA, Madeleine DeMeules BA, and Katie A. McLaughlin PhD. "Mental Health of Transgender Children Who Are Supported in Their Identities." PEDIATRICS 137, no. 3 (2016). https://doi.org/10.1542/peds.2015-3223.

[7] Russell, Stephen T., Amanda M. Pollitt, Gu Li, and Arnold H. Grossman PhD. "Chosen Name Use Is Linked to Reduced Depressive Symptoms, Suicidal Ideation, and Suicidal Behavior among Transgender Youth." Journal of Adolescent Health 63, (2018): 503-505. https://doi.org/10.1016/j.jadohealth.2018.02.003.

[8] Racine, Nicole PhD, RPsych, Brae A. McArthur PhD, RPsych, Jessica E. Cooke MSc, Rachel Eirich BA, Jenney Zhu BA, and Sheri Madigan PhD, RPsych. "Chosen Name Use Is Linked to Reduced Depressive Symptoms, Suicidal Ideation, and Suicidal Behavior among Transgender Youth." JAMA Pediatrics 175, (2021): 1142-1150. https://doi.org/10.1001/jamapediatrics.2021.2482.

Transgender children, like all children, want to belong. In 2021, when their health and well-being were threatened, North Carolina pediatricians stood up quickly and effectively in their support.

In early 2021, NCPeds convened a policy committee consisting of pediatricians, society staff, and the NCPeds lobbyist. During one of these 5:30 p.m. Wednesday discussions, the transgender legislative possibilities were discussed. During that session, no one was aware that legislators in NC had any plans to introduce transgender legislation. However, within days, legislators in our state were introducing two types of transgender legislation, and media outlets were covering the proceedings.

On March 23, 2021, House Bill 358, the legislation designed to limit transgender and intersex children's participation in athletics, was introduced at the NC legislature. AAP staff reached out to the state's already-engaged pediatricians the next day, saying it was time to take action. They were ready. AAP staff offered our leaders the policy statements and legislative testimonies of other AAP state chapters. On March 25, the NCPeds Policy Committee drafted its own statement opposing the bill, subsequently gaining approval from the society's executive committee. They consulted transgender North Carolinians and their families to ensure NCPeds appropriately addressed their perspectives and fears. They spoke with the society's lobbyists for guidance and support in clearly communicating the pediatricians' perspectives to legislators. Weeks later, when Senate Bill 514 was introduced, aiming to prohibit gender-affirming clinical care for individuals under twenty-one years of age, North Carolina's pediatricians spoke frequently with NCPeds lobbyists to clearly communicate the society's views in opposition and to communicate their readiness for action. While some of this advocacy was public, lending vocal and unequivocal support to the state's transgender youth, much of it happened quietly and behind the scenes, making sure policymakers were connected to pediatricians who could answer their questions and convince them that NC did not need either of the transgender bills.

There was no public hearing on SB514 and only one on HB358, during which transgender youth and their families and advocates gave impassioned and compelling testimonies. This was in considerable contrast to many neighboring states that saw vigorous public debate and outright passage of the bills. On April 21, 2021, General Assembly leadership announced that neither bill would be proceeding to a vote.

While various factors likely contributed to the outcome of these legislative initiatives, NCPeds infrastructure, leadership, engagement, and network of friendly like-minded organizations allowed it to react quickly, skillfully, and impactfully to communicate pediatricians' support for the state's transgender youth.

# Community-Based Coalitions: Key to Improving Child Health Outcomes

by Dave Tayloe Jr., MD, FAAP

NCPeds has developed the infrastructure to organize and conduct three open forums per year in three different locations in which pediatricians come together with a variety of health professionals, chapter staff, lobbyists, lay child advocates, and government leaders/administrators to discuss a variety of topics concerning child health and well-being. During these sessions, participants often share stories of how child advocacy plays out in their communities.

I have attended nearly every NCPeds Open Forum since 1977 and can honestly say that attending these sessions led me to establish a number of highly successful community-based coalitions.

### ADOLESCENT PREGNANCY PREVENTION

I learned about physician-led, school-based initiatives during NCPeds meetings. In 1983, after I was elected to a local board of education, our board realized that we had fifty pregnancies during a given year at our 1,300-student "city" high school. The board decided to hire a young health educator, who worked in our local health department, to work full-time at our high school. I became her supervisor and a link to the board of education. The health educator, the associate superintendent, and I had lunch in his office once a month to assure adequate support for her program. She became incredibly involved with the state's Adolescent Pregnancy Prevention Coalition, a North Carolina nonprofit organization, and established a local coalition to promote adolescent pregnancy prevention. In less than two years, our pregnancy rate at that high school dropped by nearly 50 percent, and she expanded the program to involve all students in grades five through twelve.

### CHILD ABUSE PREVENTION

NCPeds pays for the president and vice-president to attend national and district meetings of the AAP and the annual meeting of NCPeds. Therefore, I attended the 1991 AAP Annual Meeting in Boston, where Drs. Calvin Sia, Richard Krugman, and

David Olds facilitated a session on intensive home visiting. These experts convinced me that most fatal child abuse occurs very early in life and that intensive home visiting program staff, who frequently visit at-risk children's homes from birth to age five, can prevent many of these fatalities. I became convinced that our community needed an intensive home visiting program. When I returned home, I convened a group of about twenty people I knew were trying to address the needs of at-risk families in our community. We developed a parenting brochure and had regular discussions concerning the establishment of an intensive home visiting program in our community. The director of our local Head Start agency, Betsy Thigpen, arranged for us to apply for $500,000 in federal money coming through the state Department of Health and Human Services. This would allow us to establish Wayne County First Steps, a Healthy Families America project designed to train paraprofessionals to visit the homes of babies at-risk for neglect or abuse and help their families understand what is important to provide a nurturing environment that will assure optimal and safe growth and development of the children. The program was based at Head Start and carefully integrated with our Early Head Start program.

**Today, we are among the largest Reach Out and Read programs in our state.**

Our hospital gave First Steps office space adjacent to the newborn nursery so that First Steps staff could assist newborn nursery staff in administering First Steps screening instruments to all mothers during the postpartum time frame. I chaired the First Steps consortium during the fifteen-year life of the project. As Medicaid developed the Community Care of NC (CCNC) care-coordination system, Care Coordination for Children (CC4C) program, the follow-up Care Management of At-Risk Children (CMARC) initiative, and the Pregnancy Medical Home programs, and as we expanded Early Head Start to address the holistic needs of more at-risk children in the birth-to-age three group, we were able to deal with declining funding of First Steps and still provide home-visiting support for at-risk families of preschool children. Approximately 30 percent of our children live in poverty, so many are at-risk based upon social determinants of health.

## SCHOOL-BASED HEALTH SERVICES

In 1996, the Duke Endowment contacted our hospital and offered to provide $500,000 in funding to start two school-based health centers in our county because

Wayne County had the ninth most uninsured school-aged children of all the 100 counties in NC. The hospital contacted me to say they would go along with this plan if Goldsboro Pediatrics provided leadership and support. I agreed to work with the hospital on this project, based upon what I had learned about school-based health services from our pregnancy prevention program and discussions with colleagues during NCPeds Open Forum sessions.

The Duke Endowment funds enabled the launch of the Wayne Initiative for School Health (WISH). I have served as the chair of the board and medical director for WISH ever since. Today, WISH operates seven school-based health centers in three high schools, three middle schools, and one alternative school. Goldsboro Pediatrics is the overarching medical home for the more than 4,000 students served in these schools. The staff of the WISH Centers utilizes the electronic health record system of the practice. Through this program, many at-risk students not only receive traditional pediatric health services but they have access to health educators, mental health professionals, and nutritionists who come into the centers to augment the array of services offered by WISH staff. We collaborate with school-based health centers in three other counties on a psychosocial screening research project. Former chapter president and AAP board member, Dr. Jane Foy, a key contributor to the mental health initiatives of the AAP, is directing this project. Jane and I met during an NCPeds meeting more than twenty years ago.

## EARLY LITERACY

I learned about Reach Out and Read during chapter open forum meetings. In 2004, a young pediatric nurse practitioner joined our practice and convinced me that she and I could raise the money necessary (about $40,000 annually) to implement Reach Out and Read for our practice. Today, we are among the largest Reach Out and Read programs in our state. In 2013, we realized that up to 82 percent of US children in poverty were not reading at grade level when they entered fourth grade. The practice led the effort to establish Read Wayne, a coalition of service organizations dedicated to improving child outcomes. Our hospital created a video of me talking about early literacy and the importance of face-to-face parent-child interaction during the first three years of life, including reading to children more and utilizing screen-based media less. Parents and teachers were also included in this video. We staged several community forums to promote our early literacy agenda. The Wayne County Public Library director obtained grant funding through the National Library Association to hire three full-time staff to go out into the community to promote our agenda. United Way donated $600,000 to our cause so that we could establish a birth-to-age three center for up to thirty-six at-risk families in the rural southwestern region of our county where elementary reading scores are quite low. Recently, we expanded our Reach Out and Read program to include newborns through first grade and established lending libraries in various locations in our county for older children.

## SCHOOL-BASED HEPATITIS B IMMUNIZATION

In 1991, North Carolina began to offer hepatitis B vaccines to all newborns and infants according to the recommendations of the American Academy of Pediatrics. Sam Katz, MD, FAAP, was chairman of the department of pediatrics at Duke University then and was well connected at state, national, and international levels with childhood immunization developments. Dr. Katz was a regular attendee at NCPeds Open Forum meetings. I asked him why we were giving the hepatitis B vaccine to infants when we should be immunizing adolescents based on imminent risk issues. Dr. Katz replied that he did not think we could reach adolescents easily but that the infants were a captive audience for pediatricians. I argued that we could immunize adolescents by taking the vaccine to schools. (see *School-Based Hepatitis B Immunization*) He agreed to try to find grant funding so that I could pilot this idea. Dr. Katz convinced the state immunization branch to apply for Centers for Disease Control and Prevention funding to implement a school-based hepatitis B immunization pilot program in two NC counties, our rural eastern county of Wayne and the western rural county of Caldwell. The pilot involved nurses from the health department going into the elementary schools and offering hepatitis B vaccines to fourth-grade students whose parents signed release forms for the students to receive the vaccine. Seventy-five percent of the students received the vaccine. Based upon this data, the state began offering hepatitis B vaccines to all sixth-grade students and continued doing this until the babies born in 1991 reached sixth grade and therefore had already been immunized.

# Part IV

Pediatric Academicians:
Powerful Partners
Cite the Importance of
Collaboration with NCPeds

# Atrium Health Wake Forest Baptist Brenner Children's Hospital and Department of Pediatrics, Winston-Salem

by Allison McBride, MD, FAAP; Anna Miller-Fitzwater, MD, MPH, FAAP

Stating that NCPeds is an organization for pediatricians in no way captures the essence of the organization. Our experiences with NCPeds have demonstrated that this dedicated group has been brought together by their desire to be up to date on the latest in pediatric medicine and more so by their ultimate goal of improving child health. It is at an NCPeds meeting where you will see local pediatricians and academic pediatricians joining together to learn, share experiences, brainstorm new collaborative initiatives, and advocate for children.

The history of the Wake Forest University Department of Pediatrics is tightly woven with that of NCPeds. Efforts to enhance learner experience and scholarship, create progressive legislation for children, and broaden the impact of our care took root through NCPeds. Of particular significance to an academic training program, NCPeds affords our residents and junior faculty opportunities to make statewide and national connections early in their careers in ways that shape their future career paths, creating leaders that broadly and positively impact children's health for decades. Recent illustrative examples include:

- networking with state experts surrounding the successful transitions of children with medical complexity to adult care models;
- collaborating with the Forsyth County Department of Social Services to create a county-wide foster care medical home network through the Fostering Health Initiative;
- attending legislative conferences and "White Coat Wednesdays" that allow clinicians to learn how to effectively use their voices to advocate for children on a multitude of topics; and,
- successfully working with the North Carolina Department of Health and Human Services to create a government-funded $3 million health services initiative to enhance the pediatric primary care standard by promoting literacy and early relational health via expansion of the Reach Out and Read model throughout North Carolina.

NCPeds has made a tremendous impact on each of our careers, and we are proud to encourage all our trainees to become involved in the organization as they begin their pediatric careers.

# Atrium Health Levine Children's Hospital and Department of Pediatrics, Charlotte

by Amina Ahmed, MD, FAAP, FPIDS; H. Stacy Nicholson, MD, MPH, FAAP

NCPeds has a longstanding reputation as a strong state chapter of the American Academy of Pediatrics (AAP), and the children of North Carolina are fortunate to have a strong AAP chapter in their state.

The children's service line at Atrium Health is unique among North Carolina institutions focused on children. We are comprised of Levine Children's Hospital (LCH), a full-service subspecialty focused academic medical center, and our pediatric primary care division, including more than 160 pediatricians practicing in eight North Carolina counties and York County, South Carolina. Thus, we have multiple ways of contributing to and benefiting from our involvement with NCPeds.

> The active advocacy on a state, regional, and national level improves the lives of the children we serve.

Both our LCH faculty members and community pediatricians have served in key roles to help execute the work conducted by NCPeds. In this capacity, NCPeds has helped unite "town and gown" toward the common goal of advocating for children in North Carolina. Dr. J.C. Parke, the first chair of pediatrics at what was then known as Charlotte Memorial Hospital, was an avid supporter of NCPeds. Dr. Bob Schwartz, who was on faculty at the time, served as president of NCPeds from 1987–1989. Dr. Herb Clegg, representing Charlotte from Eastover Pediatrics, served as president from 2006–2008, and Dr. Karen Breach of University Pediatrics, from 2010–2012. Dr. Oliver Roddey and Dr. Edward "Ned" Martin of Eastover Pediatrics served as inaugural members of the liaison committee, a statewide NCPeds support group that today meets three times a year as the open forum.

Since then, others have served on the board and contributed to multiple committees such as the membership committee (Dr. Preeti Matkins), diversity committee (Matkins), child abuse and neglect committee (Matkins), committee on infectious disease (Amina Ahmed), adolescent health subcommittee (Matkins), and the education committee (Amina Ahmed, Candace Howell). Others have contributed as chapter immunization representatives or local media contacts. Dr. Harry Smith (Charlotte Pediatrics) was instrumental in setting up the senior physician interest group, and Dr. Andrew Shulstad (Charlotte Pediatrics) helped launch the young physician interest group.

The annual meetings have been instrumental in allowing residents to interact with pediatricians and other residents across the state. Numerous residents from LCH engaged in the poster sessions, often garnering first or second place awards. The poster sessions not only allowed them to network with pediatricians but showed the support across all academic centers for future pediatricians. The residents benefited tremendously from postgraduate year two and postgraduate year three "Resident Days," which allowed them to network with practices and pediatricians across the state as they started their job searches.

Our faculty, pediatricians, and pediatric residents benefit from the education and networking opportunities that NCPeds provides. The active advocacy on a state, regional, and national level improves the lives of the children we serve. We look forward to contributing to the future success of NCPeds!

# Maynard Children's Hospital and Brody School of Medicine Department of Pediatrics, Greenville

by Matthew R. Ledoux, MD, FAAP; Dale A. Newton, MD, FAAP; Jon Tingelstad, MD, FAAP; Chuck Willson, MD, FAAP

A strength of NCPeds continues to be the organization's emphasis on advocacy for children. With optimal health, well-being, and futures of North Carolina's children as its primary goals, the organization has gained credibility with state agencies, legislators, foundations, and other nonprofit organizations. Leaders from state agencies and legislators are frequent participants in the open forums and annual meetings, and this opportunity for dialogue has often resulted in progress toward important policies or legislation to improve child health outcomes.

NCPeds also advocates for pediatricians. Efforts directed toward enhanced implementation and payment for NC Medicaid have led to improved patient access and health delivery, with specific improvements in payment for acquiring vaccines and administering immunizations, practice management strategies, performing health supervision visits, participating in the dental health initiative to apply fluoride for young children, and even finding systemic errors in state payment systems. Improved payment positively impacts private pediatricians and also benefits our East Carolina University (ECU) general pediatric clinic practice. Besides working on improving vaccine acquisition and practice management strategies, the organization also has

145

provided implementation and guidance for the electronic medical record (EMR) and the changing role of pharmacists in health care.

NCPeds is a provider of continuing medical education and opportunities for professional development for pediatricians and other affiliated child health professionals. This is often in the form of lectures and workshops at the annual meeting or during open forums, and faculty from our department participate regularly as teachers in these venues. ECU has hosted multiple open forums throughout the years.

Like the other academic centers, ECU has historically had close ties to NCPeds. Faculty member Dr. Charles Willson was president of NCPeds from 2002-2004. Dr. Dale Newton served on the executive committee, chaired the council on political and academic affairs, and for many years, was the liaison to the North Carolina Department of Health and Human Services for the pediatric lead screening program. Dr. David Eldridge, another of our faculty, now serves in this position. Our former chairs (Drs. Jon Tingelstad and Ron Perkin) attended the open forums and annual meetings when time allowed, or would send a designee. This provided an opportunity to know and communicate with community pediatricians and to provide an academic center report to attendees.

NCPeds is especially important to the education of our residents. Through NCPeds they get to see what effective advocacy looks like. They are encouraged to attend the open forums but more commonly attend the annual meeting. That meeting includes a resident poster session, which is an opportunity for networking and academic enrichment. The resident poster session at the annual meeting was originated by Dr. Gregg Talente, and is now co-chaired by Jennifer Crotty, MD, FAAP, and a colleague from Duke University, Dr. Dan Ostrovsky. Dr. Karin Hillenbrand is currently co-chair of the education committee. NCPeds also sponsors two career days each year, one that focuses on career options and another about transitioning to either practice or fellowship. Many of our residents have attended these activities.

The partnership between NCPeds and ECU Pediatrics has been and continues to be important to both organizations. As an academic partner with NCPeds, the pediatric department at ECU pays membership dues to the society for department faculty, and we are pleased to continue to encourage faculty engagement. NCPeds has a current initiative to increase engagement with subspecialists and hospital-based physicians. We consider ourselves lucky to have a partnership with the best pediatric state organization in the nation!

# University of North Carolina Children's Hospital and Department of Pediatrics, Chapel Hill

by Stephanie D. Davis, MD, FAAP; Mike J. Steiner, MD, MPH, FAAP

The North Carolina Pediatric Society (NCPeds) has been an incredible advocate for the children and families of North Carolina. This society also has served the pediatric trainees, faculty, other physicians, and child health professionals throughout the state by providing a platform for our voices to be heard.

North Carolina's state chapter of the American Academy of Pediatrics is well known throughout the nation as an active and effective large state chapter. Throughout the decades, NCPeds has been effective in advocating for transformative work in our state regarding vaccination, Medicaid reform (multiple times), CHIP (Child Health Insurance Program), issues regarding payment for care, and child health policy.

The national reputation for state-based work also has led to a close partnership with the UNC Department of Pediatrics at many different levels. NCPeds provides an opportunity for both academic general pediatric and specialty faculty within our department to work closely with primary care providers across the state. Faculty within the UNC Department of Pediatrics have participated in several

> NCPeds has masterfully connected the community primary care providers to the academic generalists, subspecialists, and trainees.

committees, advocacy initiatives, and leadership roles within NCPeds. Additionally, we have participated in educational sessions at the annual meeting and at other times throughout the year. NCPeds has been supportive of research pursuits and projects that emanate from the academic centers in the state and the society has supported statewide research in workforce demand and community pediatric needs. These tremendous opportunities have enriched the work of all our faculty and trainees.

The NCPeds annual meeting has provided a consistent opportunity for residents and other trainees to present scholarly projects. The clinical cases and research projects are presented at poster sessions, leading to academic collaboration across the state. Trainees also have an opportunity to interact with community-based providers, which often leads to future job opportunities. NCPeds has had an important role in training our learners in advocacy and the importance of this focus in the lives of pediatricians. Most recently, the Carolinas Collaborative—which is supported by the AAP and NCPeds and which pulled together residency programs across North Carolina and South Carolina—has become one of the core aspects of our advocacy curriculum for residents in the department.

In summary, NCPeds has masterfully connected the community primary care providers to the academic generalists, subspecialists, and trainees. The partnership between the department, UNC Children's Hospital, and NCPeds has enriched the work and professional lives of faculty and trainees. More importantly, together we have been able to support our mutual goals of improving the health and well-being of children across the state of North Carolina and beyond.

## PostScript:

*A great letter/commentary on the relationship of UNC Pediatrics and NCPeds—a relationship that benefits the children and helps to support those who speak for the needs of the children in our state and beyond. As a member of the faculty, I have seen NCPeds as a separate space from UNC. It draws an individual into a world of child advocacy, not as a UNC provider but simply a person looking to help a child. These words and feelings are embedded in the letter, which I fully support.*

– Richard W. Sutherland, MD, FAAP, Pediatric Urology at UNC, member of the Executive Committee of NCPeds; *History of the Education Committee of the NC Pediatric Society (NCPeds)*

*I started work at Moses Cone five days before the 1997 NCPeds Annual Meeting, and you were one of the first people I met at the meeting. I sat with you at breakfast, and we spoke a bit about advocacy activities. During the meeting, I learned of your leadership and recognized how accomplished NCPeds was, thanks to leaders like you and the relationships forged with state officials (something neither Maryland nor Massachusetts had). Jane Foy was installed as president during that meeting, and she invited me to start a new activity for NCPeds, a Committee on Education. I was surprised one had not existed and was pleased to be asked. That Committee was my focus for several years.*

– Ken Roberts, MD, FAAP; *email to Dave Tayloe Jr., concerning how he became involved in the NC Pediatric Society after working in academic pediatrics in Maryland and Massachusetts and being involved in child advocacy efforts in those states.*

# Duke Children's Hospital and Duke Medical Center Department of Pediatrics, Durham

**by Ann M. Reed, MD**

NCPeds is a special organization that draws together an incredible community-based network of pediatricians, along with like-minded academic pediatrics partners and a variety of non-physician, child-friendly allies to assure the survival and growth of its remarkably strong traditions of advocacy successes in our state. The North Carolina Pediatric Society is an extremely effective nexus to leverage the respective strengths of each domain of pediatric practice and advocacy.

Our academic pediatricians, who come from various high quality academic centers and health systems, benefit greatly from the society and have been involved in a variety of ways, leveraging their expertise and the power of the academic infrastructure, but in a way that is locally relevant and highly impactful. NCPeds has been incredibly welcoming of our trainees, and, year after year, gives them a close-up view of what an effective state pediatric chapter can do. Examples of this are the support of our residents through invitations for White Coat Wednesdays and the Poster Session at the annual meeting, which allow residents to network with pediatricians from across the state. In addition, the advocacy sessions at the annual meeting plant the seeds of advocacy in so many.

NCPeds has been a strong supporter and promoter of opportunities to partner academic pediatricians and resources with our community-based physicians. Such opportunities include the AAP Community Access to Child Health (CATCH) program, which supports both practicing pediatricians and residents to collaborate within their communities to advance the health of all children.

I believe we are very fortunate as a state and as academic medical centers to have an organization like the North Carolina Pediatric Society be the conduit for advocacy and partnership as we all seek to improve the outcomes of all our children, their families, and their child health professionals.

# North Carolina's Academic Achievement Award, "The Big Four:" Drs. Floyd Denny Jr., Samuel Katz, Jimmy L. Simon, John Tingelstad

## THE DENNY, KATZ, SIMON, TINGELSTAD ACADEMIC SERVICE AWARD

NCPeds has witnessed the value of the collaboration of general and subspecialist pediatricians to its advocacy efforts since the beginning of its existence. In 1991, NCPeds established the Dave Tayloe Sr. Award for the Community Pediatrician of the Year. It was fitting that NCPeds create a similar award to recognize academic and subspecialist pediatricians who contribute significantly to the successful advocacy of the organization.

In 2001, President Bill Hubbard, MD, FAAP, proposed to NCPeds executive leadership an award recognizing academic achievement in research, teaching and service. The annual award first was presented in 2002 to Bob Schwartz, MD, FAAP. It celebrates the contributions from academic members who exemplify the qualities of leadership, collaboration, and prestige represented by "The Big Four" chairs of North Carolina's pediatric medical institutions. The following commentaries highlight the careers and accomplishments of the four department chairs whose names commemorate, elevate, and inspire the pursuit of academic excellence in tandem with the spirit of advocacy.

## Floyd W. Denny, MD, FAAP

In Memoriam, 1924-2001

**By Bill Hubbard, MD, FAAP; Dave Tayloe Jr., MD, FAAP**

Floyd Denny grew up in Hartsville, South Carolina, graduated from Wofford College, and then completed medical school and residency at the Vanderbilt University School of Medicine. By then, the Korean War had started, and he was ordered to active duty in the US Army. He chose to accept an assignment to Case Western Reserve University to study the role of streptococcal disease in the etiology of acute rheumatic fever with two renowned infectious disease specialists, Dr. Charles Rammelkamp and Dr. Lewis Wannamaker.

Rheumatic fever was the most common cause of heart disease in children and young adults. The team moved to Warren Air Force Base in Wyoming where young recruits were crowded into barracks, the perfect breeding ground for streptococcal disease. Here the team carried out classic research studies demonstrating that rheumatic

Dr. Denny profoundly influenced the professional careers of hundreds of future North Carolina pediatricians who aspired to emulate his principles of scholarship, intellectual honesty, and enthusiasm for our profession.

fever could be prevented by the treatment of strep throats with ten days of penicillin. Dr. Denny was the lead author of the article that won the 1954 Lasker Award and launched Dr. Denny's career in infectious disease and epidemiology.

In 1960, at the age of thirty-seven, he was selected to be the chairman for the fledgling UNC Department of Pediatrics, which at that time consisted of six faculty and twelve house staff. Under his leadership, the department grew to forty full-time faculty members, forty-four pediatric and med-peds house staff, and twenty fellows. He also developed community-based training sites in Charlotte, Greensboro, and Raleigh. Dr. Denny served as the pediatric chair until 1981.

Despite his administrative and teaching responsibilities, his passion for research never waned. He developed a productive pediatric infectious disease division of five to seven infectious disease specialists, over which he remained the driving force and chief. The division focused its research on streptococcal and mycoplasma disease, plus a lengthy longitudinal study of the epidemiology, seasonality, and symptoms of childhood viral respiratory diseases. He presented much of this published research while serving as president of the Society for Pediatric Research and the Infectious Diseases Society of America.

*Dr. Bill Hubbard, a UNC medical school and pediatric residency graduate comments: Perhaps his greatest gratification came from teaching pediatric house staff. He committed an enormous amount of his time to personal education of the pediatric residents. Every Monday, Wednesday, and Thursday at 8:30 a.m., all junior and senior residents met in Dr. Denny's office. Interns were not included. Junior residents were responsible for presenting patients who had been admitted during the previous twenty-four hours. Initially, these rounds were intimidating. Dr. Denny had high standards and expected excellence. Poorly prepared, disorganized, or incomplete presentations were sharply criticized. One didn't want to disappoint the chief.*

*Over time, residents grew comfortable, and realized how incredibly valuable these teaching hours were. We all remember how often this brilliant clinician would say, "I don't know the answer to this child's problem, but here's how I suggest we address it."*

*Dr. Denny's contributions to pediatrics and the welfare of children were recognized with multiple awards, including the Distinguished Alumnus Award from Vanderbilt University, the Outstanding Civilian Service Award from the Surgeon General of the Army, the O. Max Gardner Award from the UNC Board of Governors, and, in 1988, the NC Medal of Science from Governor James G. Martin.*

*Dr. Dave Tayloe Jr. comments: I ended up with my first choice at St. Christopher's Hospital for Children in Philadelphia, and after two years, had decided to go into general pediatrics. Knowing that I wanted to return to North Carolina, I contacted Dr. Denny, and explained to him that I needed to spend a year with a mentor like him, and asked to come back to UNC for my final year of residency. He found a way to allow me to do that. What I observed was the difference between night and day in terms of leadership in managing a department of pediatrics. It was no surprise to me when some of his residents established the Floyd W. Denny Society to honor him and nourish the traditions of Dr. Denny as chair of pediatrics for twenty years!*

*Dr. Denny profoundly influenced the professional careers of hundreds of future North Carolina pediatricians who aspired to emulate his principles of scholarship, intellectual honesty, and enthusiasm for our profession.*

## Samuel L. Katz, MD, FAAP

In Memoriam, 1927-2022

by Peter J. Morris, MD, MPH, MDiv, FAAP, FACPM; Ann M. Reed, MD; Steve Shore, MSW

NCPeds introduced the Liaison Committee concept in 1968, and it coincided with the arrival of Samuel L. Katz, MD, FAAP, the newly appointed chair of the Duke University School of Medicine Department of Pediatrics. Dr. Katz would become a frequent participant at NCPeds meetings, often as a lecturer on infectious diseases or describing the latest in vaccine development. In the commentaries on the history of North Carolina vaccine legislation and immunization programs that appear throughout this book, Dr. Katz was often front and center as a recognized and reliable advocate who brought exceptional knowledge and investigative experience with an international reputation and a presence that belied his genial nature. On multiple occasions he attended hearings at the state legislature to answer questions and to emphasize and promote vaccines.

Prior to his arrival at Duke, Dr. Katz submitted his application for membership to NCPeds with two letters of nomination: Jerome Harris, MD, FAAP, who was the pediatric chair at Duke, and Floyd Denny, MD, FAAP, pediatric chair at the University of North Carolina. Dr. Katz had an impressive medical career that started when he earned his MD at Harvard University; he then completed a co-residency at Children's Hospital Medical Center in Boston and at St. Mary's Hospital Medical School in London. He next served as a research fellow at the National Foundation for Infantile Paralysis, and was awarded the Research Career Development Award of the National Institute of Allergy and Infectious Diseases of the National Institutes of Health in 1965. From tutor to instructor to associate to assistant professor at Harvard Medical School, he was co-director of the Infectious Disease Career Training Program shared by Beth Israel Hospital and Children's Hospital Medical Center, Boston, when he took the appointment to come to North Carolina.

Dr. Katz was already active with the American Academy of Pediatrics, having served on the Committee on Infectious Diseases and having chaired the Massachusetts Chapter of the AAP's Committee on the Control of Infectious Diseases. When he arrived at Duke, he was soon contributing to the scientific meetings and the advocacy agenda of NCPeds. Throughout his tenure at Duke, Dr. Katz displayed genuine interest in his patients, faculty, and trainees, actively encouraging women and minority physicians and seeking to diversify the faculty. "Sam just had that way of making you feel like a colleague and peer—even though he was the mentor," said Peter J. Morris, MD, FAAP, MDiv, president of NCPeds from 2004-2006.

> Dr. Katz has been a stellar role model for all of us, as a clinician, as a teacher, as an investigator and as an advocate for children.

"Dr. Katz has been a stellar role model for all of us, as a clinician, as a teacher, as an investigator and as an advocate for children," said Duke Department of Pediatrics Chair Ann M. Reed, MD.

Senior pediatricians in NCPeds cordially recall that, on occasion, the department chairpersons, including Dr. Floyd Denny at UNC, Dr. Katz at Duke, Dr. Jimmy Simon at Wake Forest University, and Dr. Jon Tingelstad at East Carolina University, would sometimes travel to visit with community pediatricians or host meetings at the medical schools. Other commentaries in this book highlight the strong bonds between North Carolina's medical schools, the clerkship and residency programs, and NCPeds. This collaboration that brought academic and community practitioners together with policymakers and administrative program managers to advance children's health has been described as one of NCPeds secret weapons.

Dr. Katz was the chair of Duke Pediatrics until 1990, but he never left Duke and continued to mentor, teach, and conduct research. He expanded his role as an advocate for vaccination after experiencing firsthand the ways in which disease affects children living in resource-poor countries, notably in Africa. This work contributed to his lifelong record of advocacy and included his wife, Dr. Catherine M. Wilfert, MD, FAAP, an internationally recognized pediatric AIDS and infectious disease specialist.

The list of state, national, and international committees and organizations that Dr. Katz advised and served as a member, often as chair, illustrates the energy that he brought to any task, and accounts for the affection and esteem that NCPeds holds for "Dr. Sam" along with his family, friends and colleagues.

## Jimmy L. Simon, MD
In Memoriam, 1930-2020

by Robert Schwartz, MD, FAAP

I was president of NCPeds from 1987–89, and came to Bowman Gray School of Medicine (now Wake Forest University School of Medicine) in 1992. As president of NCPeds, I quickly learned of the important role that Jimmy Simon played in advocacy for children in North Carolina. Dr. Simon always attended the annual and quarterly meetings of NCPeds. On a rotating basis, he served as a member of the executive committee with responsibility for planning the academic program for the annual meeting. Dr. Simon was never shy about speaking up, especially on issues involving the health and welfare of children. I can recall a time when the Children's Special Health Services Program (then called the Crippled Children's Program) was planning to decrease payments to the Academic Medical Centers. Dr. Simon called me and other pediatric chairs and leaders, and said we could not and would not accept the lower payments. However, we should and would continue to provide care for those children needing medical services. It did not take long for the state of North Carolina to reinstate the previous payment levels. The fees were increased at a later time. Sara Sinal, MD, FAAP, and Mike Lawless, MD, FAAP, faculty members in general pediatrics and adolescent medicine, reported that Dr. Simon, in cooperation with the other pediatric medical school chairs, lobbied the legislature any time there was an issue affecting children, specifically Medicaid funding, traffic and vehicle safety, and immunizations.

Dr. Simon encouraged the pediatric faculty to attend and get involved in committees of NCPeds and the American Academy of Pediatrics. Jane Foy, MD, FAAP, who joined the general pediatrics faculty in 1996, reported that Dr. Simon mentored her early efforts to publish about state-level child advocacy and gave her tremendous

Dr. Simon's greatest legacy is in the area of pediatric education. He was selected as teacher of the year on six separate occasions, a record for a Wake Forest University School of Medicine faculty member.

support in seeking and serving in leadership roles in NCPeds and the American Academy of Pediatrics (AAP). He also sponsored faculty to become members of the American Board of Pediatrics.

Dr. Simon was the chair of a task force to study and write a report on the future of pediatric education. Simon rounds were held on weekdays with the pediatric residents and students. I attended a number of these sessions, and although Dr. Simon was tough and had high expectations, the residents learned to be prepared, and were proud to state that they had been "Simonized." Dr. Simon never missed grand rounds unless he was out of town, and, if he was out of town, he was attending a pediatric meeting. He was a member of the AAP Committee on Federal Government Affairs (COFGA) for many years. In his honor, the pediatric residents put on a Jimmy Simon weekend symposium and celebration after he retired. There is also a Jimmy Simon Visiting Professor Annual Lecture.

In 2001, NCPeds created an annual Academic Service Award named after the pediatric department chairpersons at that time: The Denny (Floyd Denny), Katz (Samuel Katz), Simon (Jimmy Simon), Tingelstad (Jon Tingelstad) Award. Dr. Simon's greatest legacy is in the area of pediatric education. He was selected as teacher of the year on six separate occasions, a record for a Wake Forest University School of Medicine faculty member. In 1996, he received the Joseph St. Geme Award from the Federation of Pediatric Organizations. This award represents a true measure of his impact on pediatric education. Even in retirement, he was engaged in pediatric education with student teaching, advising students and faculty, and as a reviewer for the Residency Review Committee of the Accreditation Council for Graduate Medical Education. Finally, in what Dr. Simon considered his greatest accomplishment, he was able to get a prominent Winston-Salem family to finance the Brenner Children's Hospital.

Thank you to Jane Foy, Sara Sinal, Mike Lawless, Jon Abramson, and Jimmy Simon's wife, Marilyn Simon, for help with writing this commentary.

# Jon B. Tingelstad, MD, FAAP

In Memoriam, 1935-2023

by Dale Newton, MD, FAAP; Chuck Willson, MD, FAAP

Not afraid to take on a challenge, Dr. Tingelstad was hired in 1976 as the first pediatric faculty member in the totally new medical school in Greenville, North Carolina. He was recruited by his former chair of pediatrics at Medical College of Virginia, Dr. William Laupus. Dr. Laupus had just been named dean at ECU School of Medicine (now Brody School of Medicine), and took on the additional title of chair of pediatrics. When the accrediting survey team from the Liaison Committee on Medical Education reviewed the status of the new school, they recommended that the dean should not also be a chair. Dean Laupus then initiated a national search for a department chair. Dr. Tingelstad was in the uncomfortable position of playing host to prospective chairs and aiding in recruiting them, while being under consideration for the position. On October 1, 1977, Dean Laupus enthusiastically named Dr. Tingelstad as chairman of pediatrics.

The new position was certainly challenging due to the lack of facilities, reputation, rural location, and perhaps even the school's birth from a cauldron of boiling politics. Dr. Tingelstad was qualified for his role in so many ways. With roots in North Dakota, perhaps he had more comfort in this rural setting. He attended medical school at Harvard University, followed by pediatric residency at Children's Hospital Medical Center, Boston, and University of Colorado Medical Center, Denver. Training in pediatric cardiology followed at Buffalo's Children's Hospital. He then moved to Richmond and attained associate professor status before moving to Greenville.

The challenges become more real with some examples: Housed in Ragsdale Hall on ECU's main campus, Dr. Tingelstad had to clear off his desk to provide an examination table for his first pediatric consultation. Later, he performed the first-ever pediatric heart catheterization in Eastern North Carolina. Slowly, facilities were borrowed, leased, or built as the fledgling department grew in numbers of faculty, subspecialties, and patients. Most of the new faculty, regardless of subspecialty, still had to be general pediatricians to some degree since the few faculty were providing services in clinics, wards, nursery, and even pediatric intensive care. In 1977, the first four-year class of twenty-eight medical students matriculated at East Carolina University and were followed quickly by the first pediatric residents. Combined medicine-pediatric residents joined the numbers in 1986. By that year, the faculty had increased to twenty-four. Dr. Tingelstad noted that, in recruiting, he had to be careful that faculty candidates didn't inadvertently fly to Greenville, South Carolina. By his retirement in 2000, the department consisted of forty-two pediatric faculty, sixteen divisions, and new clinical services at in-patient and out-patient locations.

In addition to being a highly effective clinician and educator, Dr. Tingelstad proved to be an able communicator, recruiter, and administrator.

In addition to being a highly effective clinician and educator, Dr. Tingelstad proved to be an able communicator, recruiter, and administrator. Beginning in 1986, the department raised funds through participation in the Children's Miracle Network Telethon. Dr. Tingelstad became a member of the board of the American Board of Pediatrics, and chaired the board in 1998. The department's annual pediatric continuing medical education course honors him by being named The Jon B. Tingelstad Conference: Practical Pediatrics. NCPeds gives an annual award to an academic member of the organization, and it is appropriately named to honor the long-time chairs: The Denny, Katz, Simon, Tingelstad Academic Achievement Award.

## NCPeds Education Committee

by Kenneth B. Roberts, MD, FAAP

I became involved in NCPeds after working in academic pediatrics in Maryland and Massachusetts. I had been involved in child advocacy efforts in those states. I started work at Moses Cone five days before the 1997 NCPeds Annual Meeting. Dave Tayloe was one of the first people I met at the meeting.

I had completed my term as the immediate past president of the Association of Pediatric Program Directors (APPD), and Jane knew about me. When she invited me to chair a new education committee, I started thinking about potential members and did not have to look far to find qualified experts: Dr. Mike Lawless, a longtime friend at Wake Forest and president of the Council on Medical Student Education in Pediatrics (COMSEP); Dr. Mike Norman, pediatric nephrologist and chair of the department of pediatrics at Carolinas Medical Center in Charlotte, whom I also knew, was on the APPD board as a councilor (a position Dr. Bob Schwartz had held ten years earlier); Dr. Gil Liu, a resident at UNC, was the sole resident representative to the pediatrics residency review committee (RRC). We were loaded in NC!

I posed ideas to Jane, such as convening the five residency program directors, their graduating and rising chief residents, and coordinators for a meeting in the spring

157

(as we had been doing in Massachusetts for several years) and convening the four medical school pediatric clerkship directors with leaders of medical student pediatric interest groups and students interested in pediatrics. She was fine with that (though I was given no budget.)

The next issue was a bit trickier: The NCPeds Annual Meeting scientific session. The chairs rotated responsibility for the session and used it to drum up business by having their faculty give presentations (generally new faculty). I had a different view and proposed that we have a practitioner representative on the committee from near each of the academic centers in the state, someone who attended grand rounds regularly. The idea was for the practitioners to identify the "best grand rounds" of the year so we could invite the speakers to share their presentations with NCPeds members statewide.

> There are lots of opportunities with a committee on education in such a phenomenal organization as NCPeds!

My sense of NCPeds is that its members deserved to have the best presentations as determined by their fellow practitioners rather than being subjected to what seemed to me largely advertising. (Please forgive my cynicism.) I was fortunate that Jon Tingelstad, chair of the department of pediatrics at the Brody School of Medicine at East Carolina University in Greenville, was fine with that, and it was his turn in the rotation to organize the education program for the annual meeting. In spite of our open discussions, I will admit that there was some lingering sentiment among the five department chairs that they would like to be able to showcase their new faculty.

Dr. Lee Gilliatt, a general practitioner in Shelby, had been running career days for residents, and he was happy to collaborate, permitting us to expand the career days from opportunities in practices to opportunities in both practice and subspecialty fellowships. It may seem like we had an ambitious agenda, especially since we had no budget. Fortunately, Dr. Jim Stockman, president and chief executive officer of the American Board of Pediatrics (ABP), based in Chapel Hill, NC, agreed to host the meeting of program directors, chief residents, and coordinators. Construction limited the first meeting to the morning only, but we chose the same day as UNC's leadership conference for residents in the afternoon for those who were interested.

The neat thing about that first meeting was that I could organize it under the auspices of NCPeds and hold it at the offices of the ABP; I knew enough about the competition over basketball, let alone concern about competition in recruitment, to recognize the value of a neutral host and a neutral site.

Over the years, we were able to continue the program directors', chief residents', and coordinators' meetings, but after I stepped down, the other pieces seemed to drift away from the committee on education (e.g., career days) or drift away entirely (clerkship directors, student leaders, and students interested in pediatrics).

Identifying topics and speakers for the annual meeting was changed in accordance with the Accreditation Council for Graduate Medical Education (ACCME) guidelines. However, when Dr. Bill Hubbard was president from 2000-02, we added a basic science presentation by a gifted researcher in the state. I was initially skeptical of how well such offerings would be received, but the presentations were mind-blowing and exciting. We were able to recruit the subspecialty surgeons for workshops and subspecialists from the various centers; those were always interesting (and sometimes contentious) as it became evident how differently individual clinical issues were addressed.

There are lots of opportunities with a committee on education in such a phenomenal organization as NCPeds!

# Why NCPeds Matters to Pediatric Surgical Subspecialists

by J. Duncan Phillips, MD, FACS, FAAP

Most pediatric surgical subspecialists belong to several professional societies associated with their specialties, such as the American College of Surgeons, the American Urological Association, or the American Association of Neurological Surgeons. Since most pediatric surgical subspecialists began their post-graduate education in the "adult" part of their specialty and subsequently did pediatric-specific fellowship training, this makes sense. Why, then, should a pediatric surgical subspecialist join NCPeds? There are at least eight good reasons:

    **1. Size.** Because the American Academy of Pediatrics (AAP) has 67,000 members, including 45,000 board-certified physicians, the number of doctors represented is greater than almost any pediatric specialty medical society. As a result, its *voice*—in Washington, DC, in various state capitols, and in the public—is *louder* than most surgical societies, which may have only a few thousand members. Plus, North Carolina state legislators listen to NCPeds.

**2. Children.** Almost all of us strive (or want to strive) to have a special place in our hearts and souls for kids. We place children on a pedestal, hoping to protect them. Because the AAP advocates, in general, for children rather than for doctors, legislators, and others, they tend to view the AAP's efforts as more "pure" and less self-serving than some other medical/surgical organizations. NCPeds is, in general, seen as placing children above everyone else.

**3. Concern with Government Funding and Access to Care.** Many children live in conditions of poverty, and therefore, more than 50 percent of US children require government assistance if they are to receive a variety of needed health and human services. In addition, large numbers of poor immigrant children enter our nation and state every week. Therefore, pediatricians and pediatric surgical subspecialists have a special interest in making sure that health programs function as efficiently as possible so at-risk children have access to necessary services. NCPeds has a lengthy track record of working with the NC legislature, including long-standing, persistent, and successful efforts to raise Medicaid payment rates for physicians to parity with Medicare.

**4. Inclusion.** Pediatricians realize that pediatric surgical subspecialists come from varied backgrounds and training. For example, in most academic medical centers (and medical schools), there may be one department of pediatrics, but surgeons who care for kids may come from a multitude of separate, diverse departments, including surgery, urology, ophthalmology, neurosurgery, and orthopedics. The AAP encourages surgeons from these various disciplines to work together with pediatricians on behalf of children. For decades, NCPeds has had at least one pediatric surgical subspecialist on its board of directors, helping guide policy and develop educational programs for attendees of society meetings.

**5. Education of the Specialist.** Because pediatric surgical specialists approach the care of kids from such different backgrounds, they are frequently unaware of the day-to-day struggles of the typical practicing pediatrician. Immunizations, well-child visits, developmental assessments, and other critically important aspects of basic pediatric care are typically ignored during surgical training, leaving the surgical subspecialist easily confused about the best ways to interact with their colleagues in pediatrics. NCPeds teaches surgeons what is important to pediatricians.

**6. Education of the Pediatrician.** Pediatricians are generally hungry for knowledge regarding optimal ways to diagnose and treat pediatric conditions that may require surgical intervention, such as acute appendicitis and undescended testes. NCPeds offers educational programs for its membership, guided by pediatric surgical specialists. Because pediatricians often lead the way in the development of cost-efficient and cost-conscious protocols, surgical specialists are especially encouraged to share tips and tricks for diagnosis and treatment involving such principles.

7. **Collaboration.** As clearly documented in the 1960s and 1970s with the establishment of pediatric oncology collaborations such as the Children's Cancer Study Group (CCSG) and the Pediatric Oncology Group (POG), pediatricians and pediatric surgical subspecialists can work together, and dramatically change outcomes with pediatric cancer survival rates rising about 8 percent during each decade, beginning almost to the day that those groups came into existence. Unlike many care providers, pediatricians and pediatric surgical subspecialists in NCPeds "play well together in the sandbox."

8. **Subspecialty Sections.** Since the AAP long ago recognized that physicians other than pediatricians are typically involved frequently in the care of children, the organization developed multiple subspecialty sections, encouraging input from non-pediatricians and the ability to become official fellows of the AAP. Indeed, the surgical section of the AAP was actually established before the American Pediatric Surgical Association (APSA). Such input from non-pediatricians remains valuable to this day.

I have been a proud NCPeds member since moving to North Carolina in 1999, and I encourage my surgical subspecialist colleagues to do the same.

# Leadership and Pediatric Surgical Subspecialists

by Timothy P. Bukowski, MD, FACS, FAAP

NCPeds has had more impact on the care and well-being of all the children in NC than any other organization. It is NCPeds that I feel provides an umbrella organization under which the multiple separate pediatric groups can come together in this state, especially in working with the legislature to improve the outcomes of children.

When I moved here in 1995 as the full-time pediatric urologist at the University of North Carolina (UNC), the North Carolina Children's Hospital was a hospital within a hospital like the systems at Duke University, Charlotte, and Wake Forest University. I came from a private free-standing pediatric hospital, Children's Hospital of Michigan, with its own board of directors, executive health care team consisting of the pediatric specialty department chairs, and a board of visitors responsible for all the fundraising at the hospital. Most of the complex pediatric patients from throughout the state were funneled there for care (or at Motts Children's in Ann Arbor). Therefore, there was a direct line item in the state budget for children's care in Michigan that addressed funding for both children's hospitals. Because Children's Hospital of Michigan was an independent hospital, there was complete control of children's services, compared to what I saw in North Carolina's university centers. Children's services were secondary considerations in the North Carolina university system. I felt as though I was a stepchild straddling pediatric surgery and the urology division and had no voice in the administration. I felt there was very little communication among specialists at different hospitals in the state.

So, in October 1998, I spoke to Dr. Jane Foy, president of NCPeds, and we decided to start a surgical subspecialty section of NCPeds. The goal was to get all children's health care providers under one tent. There were approximately 1,000 member pediatricians at that time. In NCPeds, there was already a section for pediatric medical subspecialists. As surgical subspecialists, we became pediatrics subspecialists after training in our main surgical area. Pediatric radiologists and anesthesiologists shared our plight. The AAP has sections of the various surgical subspecialties that meet at the time of the annual AAP meeting in October, but there were not any statewide subspecialty groups meeting at NCPeds.

With help from NCPeds Membership Chair Dr. Dave Williams and Executive Director Dave Rock, we reached out to the pediatric program directors around the state and developed a list of surgical specialists. We surveyed specialists to develop a list of problems with which we needed the help of NCPeds. We had our inaugural meeting at the NCPeds Open Forum in February 2000. By that time, Steve Shore had taken over as executive director and helped us host a simultaneous meeting.

We accumulated a list of sixty-seven pediatric surgical subspecialists; of these, twenty-four were listed as members of NCPeds, and eleven came to the winter 2000 open forum. Pediatric surgeon Dr. Duncan Phillips had just moved to North Carolina and recounted how at Los Angeles Children's Hospital, their group of pediatric surgical subspecialists had its own lobbyist in Sacramento to address problems with medical fees for surgeons. Patients in California had limited access to specialists because of poor reimbursement, and this delayed care for children until problems developed that were severe and very difficult to address. Lobbying worked. Fees went up, and care was improved. He saw firsthand how a group of concerned individuals could change legislative agendas.

We discussed the fact that our group of specialists in NC were spread out among different university organizations, so it might be better to build something under the NCPeds, especially since NCPeds had effectively lobbied for childhood immunization reform, Medicaid improvements, and were helping guide the new

It is NCPeds that I feel provides an umbrella organization under which the multiple separate pediatric groups can come together in this state, especially in working with the legislature to improve the outcomes of children.

Health Choice program (Children's Health Insurance Program). We pledged that we would provide speakers for NCPeds members with educational materials and make sure they could contact us easily. We would support and complement educational events at the annual meetings (surgical specialist workshops) and assist in identifying gaps in pediatric surgical subspecialty care where children do not have access to necessary services.

Some of these situations revealed a need for legislative support for Medicaid (e.g., vision screening). We recommended that NCPeds include all the surgical specialist members in its member roster and allow specialists a position on the executive committee.

One of the things I remember from the open forum was learning about the creation of the North Carolina Health Choice (NCHC) Child Health Insurance Program (CHIP), which made it possible for almost all children in North Carolina to have affordable health insurance. Dr. David Bruton, Secretary of NC DHHS, gave an overview and proposed filling in the last gap by letting families above the income ceiling for NCHC buy into the system at a graduated monthly premium. The goal was to make Medicaid and NCHC seamless and to allow the uninsured an option to buy into NCHC. I thought it was great that NCPeds had a voice in the process of figuring out how to use the federal CHIP dollars efficiently.

We sent out sixty-five specialist surveys, and thirteen were sent back. The surveys revealed that the specialists were mostly interested in being more involved in the annual meeting, with opportunities to meet pediatricians. Some were interested in AMA Current Procedural Terminology (CPT) code changes, but that discussion seemed more appropriate at the national level since the AAP and AMA develop child-relevant CPT codes.

During the 2000 annual meeting in Myrtle Beach, the surgical specialists provided a "Surgical Pearls" workshop session that was very well attended. The precedent was set to have a surgical workshop at the annual meeting for the foreseeable future. Drs. Tim Weiner, Duncan Phillips, and John Weiner supervised the sessions.

The strength of the pediatric practices in North Carolina is directly related to the honest and fair input NCPeds leadership provides for NC Medicaid administrators, prepaid health plan medical directors, legislators, the secretary of Health and Human Services, and the governor.

In 2002, I started a solo pediatric urology private practice in Raleigh, operating mostly at Wake Med and taking calls with the general urologists. My practice grew very quickly, and soon I hired a nurse practitioner to care for my patients on my operating room days. This private practice business gave me more imperative to involve myself in NCPeds because of how directly my financial situation was linked to Medicaid/NC Health Choice payments. As reflected by state data, approximately 45 percent of my patients were covered by Medicaid. Therefore, Medicaid payment had to become a critical issue for me if I wanted to be able to provide care for these patients. I probably could have figured out a way to see only privately insured patients, but I felt it important to care for anyone who was referred to me. Although the Medicaid disproportionate share (DSH) federal payments helped fill gaps at the teaching hospitals for Medicaid and uninsured care, as a private practitioner, I did not receive any form of DSH payment. Fortunately, NCPeds worked with the state to develop Community Care of NC (CCNC) as the physician-directed management organization for Medicaid. Recipients were enrolled annually into CCNC, thanks to NCPeds efforts.

One of the joys of the NCPeds annual meeting has always been interacting with general pediatricians, to meet the faces of those with whom I have shared patients. "Curbside consulting" is also easier during the meetings since most community pediatricians rarely round at hospitals.

The institution of the resident research poster presentations gave me an opportunity to participate as a reviewer, and I was able to learn of general topics and meet the next generation of pediatricians. I feel fortunate to participate, as it builds community, and community maximizes communication and minimizes things that get in the way of patient care, like bias.

The strength of the pediatric practices in North Carolina is directly related to the honest and fair input NCPeds leadership provides for NC Medicaid administrators, prepaid health plan medical directors, legislators, the secretary of Health and Human Services, and the governor. While in other states, a couple of major children's hospitals may play important roles in state-based legislation, it is the selfless determination of NCPeds to improve the care of children and, by extension, the economic viability of their providers. All the NCPeds leaders have been and are incredible people, and there are just too many to name them all. As with sports, the other team is not going to make it easy to get to the goal line, but as history has proven, NCPeds has always found a way to bring the ball over.

## Advocating for Children by Bolstering the Pediatric Workforce

by Julie Story Byerley, MD, MPH

While most of the work of advocacy in pediatrics is focused on the children and their needs, it is also important to continually build and prepare the workforce of pediatricians and others who will continue the work of advocacy into the future. Medical education requires such a long training pathway that preparing a workforce of pediatricians to advocate as professionals can take a decade or more. To diversify the workforce as needed to advance equity and reduce health disparities, we must inspire a diverse group of young people into careers as pediatricians and ideally help them along the pipeline to succeed in this work.

A strength of NCPeds is how it partners with the medical schools in our state, allowing medical educators to share ideas across schools and deliver programs for large groups of learners. In the last twenty years, NCPeds has facilitated:

- the advertising of pipeline programs into careers in medicine;
- pediatric clerkship directors working together to inspire the choice of pediatric residency training for students;
- career days to help residents advance their training, especially with respect to underserved geographic locations and needed subspecialties; and
- events for young physicians just out of training to engage with NCPeds to add advocacy to their portfolio of work.

Each of these activities helps better prepare the workforce to advocate for the needs of children.

Faculty responsible for pediatric residency curricula often meet in person at the annual meeting of NCPeds. This allows us to share ideas and build relationships unique to our state. Then, at the national meetings of the Council on Medical

Student Education in Pediatrics (COMSEP) or the Association of American Medical Colleges (AAMC), we build upon the established relationships to further our work. This informal relationship-building cultivated by NCPeds pays off as we encourage graduates of our medical schools to explore the training programs in our state, allowing us to develop and keep good doctors in North Carolina.

The faculty responsible for pediatric residency training similarly are convened through NCPeds. Residency program directors collaborate to host pediatric career days for trainees twice each year—one focused on junior residents considering career choices and a later one focused on senior residents looking for jobs. These meetings allow the training programs to share resources, allow the residents in our state's five different programs to meet, and allow NCPeds to present programs that emphasize the importance of advocacy during careers while residents explore possibilities for their futures. In this setting, we can also encourage pediatric residents to consider pediatric subspecialties that are in short supply in our state. NCPeds has a strong reputation among the academic programs in NC and we look forward to collaborations that connect us to real world pediatrics outside of the ivory tower and also inspire learners into careers that affect the lives of the patients and populations we together serve.

# Engaging Medical Students and Residents for Advocacy

by Steve Shore, MSW

NCPeds executive leadership and general membership activities include a history of working with all of North Carolina's medical schools to address pediatric residents' and medical students' needs. Most often, this collaboration has led to arrangements for a panel of practicing pediatricians and a second panel of current residents to meet on the same day to conduct a general dialogue with medical students about career paths in pediatrics, descriptions of the calendar, the process for residency applications and visits, and special events geared to current advocacy topics.

During the extended health care reform debate in the US Congress from 2009–10, NCPeds leaders and the executive director visited North Carolina medical schools to report on emerging concepts in the proposed Patient Protection and Affordable Care Act. Following its enactment by Congress in March 2010, the focus changed to interpreting the key pediatric provisions in the new law. Student pediatric interest groups also contacted NCPeds office staff to obtain information about prospective pediatric advocacy projects and to help establish contact with child advocacy organizations. Another advocacy experience arranged by NCPeds executive directors matches a medical student with a specific child advocacy organization or arranges

We look forward to collaborations that connect us to real world pediatrics outside of the ivory tower and also inspire learners into careers that affect the lives of the patients and populations we together serve.

for a student to shadow a legislator or child health professional. Examples of medical student interest group projects include:

- volunteering with the NCPeds Covering Kids and Families projects and staffing application enrollment workshops for families with eligible children for Medicaid or the Children's Health Insurance Program (CHIP);
- participating in Student Action with Farmworkers, Make-A-Wish Foundation, The Covenant with North Carolina's Children—an association of child-related organizations from foster care to education to health care; and
- learning about the work of NC Child (formerly the North Carolina Child Advocacy Institute), a policy research and development agency.

When nonprofit organizations began to adopt electronic communications in the early 2000s, medical students connected to the medical school pediatric interest groups were given the option to receive all of the messaging from NCPeds about advocacy and membership meetings and were invited to attend executive leadership meetings. NCPeds leaders, present and past, have made grand rounds presentations over many years at pediatric residency programs. The executive directors have also been frequent speakers on direct advocacy initiatives.

When the Accreditation Council on Graduate Medical Education made advocacy education a core requirement for residency programs affiliated with the American Board of Medical Specialties, the American Board of Pediatrics and the American Academy of Pediatrics worked together to promote resident advocacy. One of the primary means for this activity occurred through the state chapters of the academy. North Carolina's pediatric residents were given dues-free memberships in NCPeds, were invited to attend the regional open forums without fees, and were given a special reduced rate to attend the annual meeting. The annual conference included a resident poster competition with prizes that grew from twenty-five posters entered to nearly 100 in a few years' time. The poster competition is regarded as a highlight of the annual meeting.

North Carolina started a conference on recruitment and practice management in the 1990s to enable residents to make direct contact with practices in the state. This evolved for a few years into a primary-care-focused conference with a second specialty-focused conference. Over the past decade, this arrangement has become a program year two (PGY2) conference and a program year three (PGY3) emphasizing primary care and specialty options with additional topics like negotiating compensation and contracts. Each conference includes updates on current advocacy topics in the legislative session or negotiations with private and public agencies.

NCPeds joined with the NC Medical Society in 2009 as a co-host of "White Coat Wednesdays" to encourage physicians to come to the state capitol to engage with legislators and administrative personnel. Medical white coats make a good visual to emphasize the importance of legislators consulting with the medical community and appropriate specialty groups on bills and policies designed to improve public health. NCPeds continues to be a leader in this advocacy-focused event, with residents from all of the state's medical schools invited to participate with community and academic pediatricians.

Chief residents have participated in NCPeds executive leadership meetings for many years. NCPeds executive directors have frequently arranged for residents to work directly as interns for members of the General Assembly. Other nonprofit organizations have offered similar internship opportunities.

When NCPeds received a corporate charter for its charitable foundation in 1999, the first grant awarded from a North Carolina philanthropy was titled "A Child Advocacy Initiative" for students and residents from the business, law, and medical schools at Wake Forest University. The objectives were to educate future practitioners about health policy, political processes, local and state government affairs, and current child health issues.

Dr. Jane Foy, NCPeds president for the years 1998–2000, wrote a curriculum for the activities arranged under the auspices of the grant. When the grant expired in 2001, Dr. Foy folded the child advocacy curriculum into a comprehensive community pediatric experience for Wake Forest residents and shared the curriculum with the American Academy of Pediatrics for adoption and modification in other settings. Dr. Foy and the executive director met with each of the advocacy coordinators at the five teaching and residency programs in North Carolina to explore and share lessons learned from the initiative.

During the COVID-19 pandemic, NCPeds pivoted to virtual White Coat Wednesday events coordinated by their contracted lobbyists. Leaders organized a number of online meetings that included residents, pediatricians, legislative delegations, and panels of key legislative leaders who shared insights about health policy and bills under consideration. Legislative topics were identified in advance so that residents and members could be prepared with on-point questions and recommendations.

NCPeds has supported Community Access to Child Health or CATCH grants from the American Academy of Pediatrics for individual pediatric residents and joint projects. Some of these have made advocacy the theme for securing policy change. There are five examples of North Carolina pediatric residents' CATCH grant projects in the appendix.

# Part V

## The Here and Now

# Advocacy During the Pandemic and Medicaid Transformation

**by Christoph Diasio, MD, FAAP**

I was eager to be president of NCPeds during the change from our award-winning Medicaid direct program to private insurance "managed" Medicaid because I had experience with the difficulties of managed Medicaid in another state and wanted to do what I could to make the system work as well as possible for the children, families, and child health professionals of North Carolina. I didn't anticipate that we would have to fight a killer global pandemic of COVID-19, as well as battle misinformation and disinformation at the same time! I have developed a deep and profound appreciation for the value NCPeds has and the depth and skill of our staff, in particular our executive director Elizabeth Hudgins. I already consider the privilege of leading NCPeds as the highlight of my professional career.

## KEY OVERARCHING STRATEGIES

**Solution Shares:** Early in the pandemic, NCPeds started weekly half-hour solution shares, where any member of NCPeds could join a call with fellow pediatricians and practice managers to discuss any problems they were having and potential solutions. At first, they were by conference call, then switched to Zoom video conferencing. Every Tuesday, about twenty-five to sixty pediatricians join a quick call at 5:30 p.m. to talk about everything from how practices handle physical distancing to telehealth to COVID-19 vaccination to WIC during COVID-19 to Medicaid reform. We have occasional guests, such as leadership from the Division of Public Health or North Carolina pediatrician Dr. Kathy Poehling, who serves on the Advisory Committee on Immunization Practice (ACIP) for the Centers for Disease Control (CDC).

**Membership Survey:** In Spring of 2020, NCPeds partnered with the NC Academy of Family Physicians to survey our practicing primary care members to determine their top needs around such issues as fiscal relief, access to personal protective equipment (PPE), and other issues.

Fiscal strain was the top concern for the 753 responding primary care providers, with 87 percent (92 percent of independent practitioners) reporting significant fiscal pressures. Nearly two-thirds reported at least a 40 percent drop in patient volume.

**Navigating COVID-19 Calls:** We partnered with primary care allies—Community Care of NC (CCNC), NC Academy of Family Physicians (NCAFP), NC Area Health Education Centers (NC AHEC), and NC Psychiatry Association (NCPA)— to plan and promote first weekly, and then monthly, "Navigating COVID-19" calls.

So far, we have held twenty-one learning sessions that have averaged more than 100 attendees each.

**Dedicated Web Pages:** NCPeds has created a number of dedicated web pages on topics including COVID-19 vaccines, other COVID-19 resources, Medicaid reform, routine childhood vaccine promotions, and more.

**Regular Member Communication:** Early in the pandemic, NCPeds provided breaking COVID-19 updates on an almost daily basis. Communication is now at a more regular cadence of Tuesday "COVID-19 Updates" and Friday "Weekly Wraps" on other topics. COVID-19 updates are focused more on practicing pediatricians. Also, we added anyone (member or not) who wanted the information to assure anyone who needed pediatric COVID-19 information had access. This email is sent to about 2,100 people and has an open rate of 33 to 36 percent.

Targets for weekly updates include practicing and retired pediatricians, residents, mid-levels, practice managers and staff, allies (such as child advocates), and a myriad of others. It is sent to 2,600 people with an open rate ranging from 31 to 33 percent.

**Deep Engagement about Medicaid Transformation in North Carolina:** In 2015, the NC General Assembly mandated that the state switch to managed care for Medicaid. Starting July 1, 2021, North Carolina went from one Medicaid payer and one CHIP payer to five different managed care plans, with separate Medicaid and CHIP policies while maintaining "traditional (or Direct)" Medicaid and CHIP for some high-need children (such as those with intellectual delays and disabilities or children in foster care). Some children now receive mental health services through managed care while others stay in one of the six regional systems, called LMEs (local management entities). Plans did not start paying practices until well into July and some into August.

Often, the amounts are incorrect or payments for basic services—such as vaccination, especially for CHIP children—are denied. The mechanics of getting paid can be challenging, relating to National Provider Identity (NPI), provider taxonomy, credentialing problems, banking issues, and more. NCPeds has submitted more than forty sets of comments about the transformation, and enjoys three regular monthly meetings with leadership at NC Medicaid.

NCPeds also has representation on key groups, such as the technical advisory group and the group developing the Fostering Care Plan. We also have strong relationships with the chief medical officers (CMOs) for the five insurance plans that are directing Medicaid and have been in regular contact for troubleshooting, including linking plan administrators with practices to help identify key strategies for problem resolution.

When the COVID-19 vaccine first became available for health care providers, NCPeds worked to link pediatricians and staff in independent practice with available vaccines.

**TARGETED ACTIVITIES AND RESULTS**

## Immunizations

**All vaccines:** NCPeds has shared a number of vaccine promotion resources, including AAP social media campaign materials, with membership via weekly emails and our website. We've shared vaccine promotion messages on Twitter and Facebook. NCPeds served on the steering committee for Keeping Kids Well, an NC Medicaid funded initiative led by NC AHEC and CCNC to help provide practices support for getting children in for well-child visits and vaccinations. We also shared a variety of"back to school vaccine resources. Finally, we joined with NCAFP on a project with Pfizer promoting radio Public Service Announcements (PSAs) encouraging parents to bring their children in for all vaccines. These PSAs were recorded in both English (by a family physician) and in Spanish (by a pediatrician) and placed in a wide variety of markets.

**COVID-19 Vaccine:** When the COVID-19 vaccine first became available for health care providers, NCPeds worked to link pediatricians and staff in independent practice with available vaccines. As NCPeds president, I became a "cheerleader" encouraging pediatricians to vaccinate parents and grandparents in addition to age-eligible children and provided one-on-one technical assistance in addition to media efforts, including a key op-ed and multiple media appearances/quotes. Solution shares offer a strong opportunity for members to support and advance COVID-19 vaccination. Additionally, multiple navigating COVID-19 calls focused on the mechanics of administering COVID-19 vaccines at the practice level, including the importance and "how to" for using an equity lens in administration strategy. With the assistance of Dr. Graham Barden, we negotiated a special "free delivery" rate for NCPeds members seeking to buy a super-cold freezer for storage of Pfizer COVID-19 vaccines. Using an equity lens, the NC Immunization Branch identifies regions of the state with high need and/or low vaccination rates, and NCPeds does individualized outreach and warm hand-offs to practices in those areas to help them become COVID-19 vaccinators. We have informed and promoted billing and coding for vaccine administration, including a special Medicaid code paying close to forty dollars for each counseling session for COVID-19 vaccination, even if it takes multiple sessions to help overcome hesitancy.

We've offered our solution shares "pearls of wisdom" for "fast focus groups" to the Division of Public Health to help inform system improvements, such as addressing burdensome administrative requirements. Centers for Disease Control ACIP member Dr. Kathy Poehling has been a guest on solution share twice to share updates on the COVID-19 vaccine for children.

As a result of the work of our members, pediatric practices are leading the way on COVID-19 vaccination in NC. According to our Division of Public Health, on July 21, 2021, there were a total of 676 North Carolina practices activated in the federal COVID-19 Vaccine Management System (CVMS) and 468 practices providing COVID-19 vaccines. We estimate this to be 18 percent of all practices in the state to be activated, and 12 percent vaccinating. Within that, the pediatric practices are leading the way, with 52 percent activated and 34 percent vaccinating.

**Flu Vaccine:** Given the delay often experienced by Vaccines for Children (VFC) sites receiving and distributing flu vaccines, NCPeds advocated strongly for a "two-way trade" with flu and other vaccines. Physicians who participate in VFC receive "free" vaccines through the federal-state VFC partnership for all Medicaid, uninsured, and underinsured children. Physicians purchase private sector vaccines for children who have health insurance that covers physician costs for giving the vaccines. Traditionally, physicians could not mix and match VFC and private-purchase vaccines. During COVID-19, the NC Department of Health and Human Services (DHHS) allowed physicians to give either a private or VFC vaccine to any child, as long as the physicians "pay back" the vaccines from the appropriate source during the fiscal year. This prevents patients from being sent home unvaccinated because the practice is out of stock of private purchase or VFC vaccine. You can give what you have in the fridge and swap the vaccine later. Representing NCPeds as president, I took on the role of helping create many of the training materials for this program. The NCPeds website and materials were used by pediatricians and other partners, such as AHEC and CCNC. Unfortunately, we do not yet have data on how flu vaccination of children in 2020-21 compared to previous years or other states.

**Teen Vaccines:** NCPeds joined NCAFP and the Division of Public Health to promote teen vaccines in July, when year-round school starts in North Carolina. In both 2020 and 2021, the governor declared July to be Adolescent Immunization Awareness Month, and we used this as a springboard to promote vaccinations via our public media sources and social media linkages. In 2020, North Carolina finished phasing in a twelfth grade meningitis vaccine (MCV4) requirement that NCPeds promoted via social media and weekly emails.

## Financial and Other Supports for Practices

**Member Education on Paycheck Protection Program (PPP):** Since fiscal concerns were one of the top troubles indicated by members, we sent out regular communications on PPP resources, including from AAP. One of our best-attended navigating COVID-19 sessions was on this topic. Members also shared tips via the solution share.

**Individualized Support for Members Excluded from Federal Fiscal Relief:** With AAP support, we helped provide individual support to the dozen or so practices that received a small amount of Medicare relief and were thus initially barred from receiving federal Medicaid relief through PPP. We provided one-to-one prompts on deadlines, etc.

**Increased Medicaid Payments:** As the COVID-19 pandemic proceeded, we shared our survey results showing major threats to cash flow in primary care practices with staff at NC Medicaid. One of their responses was to double the per member per month management fee (from $2.50 to $5.00) paid to practices for each Medicaid patient in a medical home; these payments were originally incorporated into the Community Care of NC medical home program to entice physicians to expand office hours to eliminate unnecessary hospital emergency department visits by patients and to work with Medicaid to avoid prescription

> As a result of the work of our members, pediatric practices are leading the way on COVID-19 vaccination in North Carolina.

of expensive pharmaceuticals when there are less expensive effective options. The increased rates during the pandemic were intended to support additional costs to practices such as developing telehealth capacity, covering increased PPE costs, and supporting staff. Practices consistently cite this as one of the key supports helping them stay afloat during the pandemic, especially since this money was sent to practices even when their visit volume dropped precipitously due to the lockdown, when families were told to stay home and to not go out to prevent infection and transmission of COVID-19. This support remains in place currently. Another key support was the 2019 increase for Medicaid to 100 percent of Medicare for primary care services.

**One Time Increase from Blue Cross Blue Shield:** We shared our survey results with Blue Cross NC and urged them to support practices in a way to help make them whole given the decline in volume. They created an Accelerate to Value Program which paid providers (who agreed to consider moving to value-based payments) a sum in 2020 to help them "true up" to 2019 payment levels.

**Support on Personal Protective Equipment:** Our joint survey with NCAFP showed that challenges getting PPE was a top concern for practices. Through involvement on various ad hoc committees, we helped modify and streamline the PPE distribution methodologies so that more independent practices could get more of the protective gear they needed. We also met jointly with the secretary of NC DHHS, NC Medical Society and NC Academy of Family Physicians to further elevate this issue.

**Navigating the Mechanics of Keeping Patients Safe During COVID-19:** Our weekly solution shares were a most valuable forum for members to share ideas ranging from using the parking lot to provide care to office cleaning routines to ventilation. Topics for navigating COVID-19 calls included office readiness, testing, and other topics of interest.

**Desktop CME (Continuing Medical Education) and Other Education:** NCPeds has offered a number of "desktop CME" options so members can fulfill CME requirements remotely on their own schedules. Our most popular offering (128 and counting) was pediatric specific options related to NC Medical Board-required opioid CME. Other sessions have ranged from media training to career fairs to yoga to self-care.

**COVID-19 Mask Battles:** A major political fight was waged over whether children should wear masks in schools when over half of the state's public schools adopted mask-optional policies. At the urging of several members, especially Dr. Teresa Forest, an open letter was sent by NCPeds to all the school boards. This letter reviewed the science and made a strong case for children to wear masks at school so they could stay in school rather than to be sent home post-exposure to COVID-19. This letter was picked up and run in a number of newspapers, and representing NCPeds, I did interviews on local NC TV news stations about the case for vaccines and masking. These efforts helped increase the number of public school districts requiring masking to nearly 100 percent.

## Telehealth

**Educating Members:** We provided telehealth education to members in a variety of formats. One navigating COVID-19 session focused on how to use telehealth encounters that had already been completed to qualify for Part IV of Maintenance of Certification for the American Board of Pediatrics (MOC-4). Our virtual Annual Meeting included a learning segment on telehealth that offered both CME and MOC-2. We shared telehealth education opportunities from a number of other

Our weekly solution shares were a most valuable forum for members to share ideas ranging from using the parking lot to provide care to office cleaning routines to ventilation.

organizations with members. "Tips of the trade" were also shared on solution shares. Weekly communications included new telehealth platforms, guidance, and flexibilities as they were announced.

**Creating Customizable Social Media Templates:** We created social media graphics designed to appeal to a diverse population so that practices could modify these to include their practice name for use on Facebook and Twitter. This helped to promote their practice's use of telehealth.

**Promoting Broadband:** We helped connect members and communities with grant opportunities to improve broadband. We shared information through various channels on special Wi-Fi hotspots and other resources. We served on a number of committees working to improve broadband access, noting the importance of an equity lens.

**Informing Policy Discussions:** NCPeds staff served on a number of telehealth workgroups in the state, helping to raise concerns about equity, especially around race and rural access.

**Working with Commercial Insurance:** Members expressed frustration that patients were charged higher copays to see their medical home pediatrician via telehealth than to see a remote telehealth doctor on contract with an insurance company. NCPeds met with United Health Care, which modified its policies and changed call center scripts to assure that patients knew they could call their medical home pediatricians.

### Keeping Medicaid and CHIP Access Strong

**Newborn Care:** Under Medicaid transformation guidelines, the original state policy was that newborns would be covered on the same Prepaid Health Plan (PHP) as their mothers. This could put babies at jeopardy if no pediatricians in the area took the same plan as the mother. It would also be problematic for pediatricians providing patient care services in newborn nurseries if they were not signed up with all five PHP's. NCPeds' persistent education of DHHS staff and PHP chief medical officers as to the impact of this policy helped result in a change that allows a provider to be paid by any plan at in-network rates during the first ninety days after birth. In North Carolina, the majority of births are to mothers with Medicaid.

**Payment:** The department was only going to test one or two claims for a handful of practices before "go-live" was scheduled to occur in Medicaid transformation. Our president insisted that all plans test approximately forty claims. Four out of the five PHPs eventually responded. This testing indicated substantial payment/claims-filing problems, especially relating to vaccine payments and especially for children covered by CHIP (who do not qualify for VFC in NC). Some improvements were made prior to going live. NCPeds continues to monitor payment issues via our robust practice manager Listserv and to work with plan CMOs to troubleshoot issues ranging from no payments to wrong payments to policies that do not align with state policy.

**Network Adequacy:** Tens of thousands of children have been auto-assigned to PHPs that do not have any contracts with hospitals within a one-hour drive of their homes. NCPeds is providing support to practices to help make it easier for families who want to switch PHPs to make those changes so that all children will have access to hospital care if needed. We also continue to emphasize the importance of universal access to pediatric subspecialists, knowing that some of our academic centers do not have all types of pediatric subspecialists due to major shortages of these subspecialists in our state.

**Panels:** NCPeds worked to assess how many patients currently assigned to a practice would likely be assigned to that same practice in Medicaid transformation. As a result of that work, the system was modified so more patients could stay in their medical homes. Additionally, I performed an analysis on the current panel in my own practice prior to go-live, pointing to a programming error with one plan that was able to be fixed ahead of go-live so that more children were correctly assigned to their regular primary care doctor at launch.

**Early Periodic Screening, Diagnosis, and Treatment (EPSDT) protections:** Initially, EPSDT-covered services would be subject to "Pay and Chase." The NCPeds Pediatric Council helped educate the department about the negative consequences of such a policy. Since go-live, we have helped rectify not paying for lead screening, not paying for certain oral health services, and other EPSDT protected services. We are still working on a myriad of other issues, including vaccine product and administration.

## Medicaid Reform

NC moved to private insurance plan-directed managed care on July 1, 2021. NCPeds has been active in identifying and troubleshooting problems. Some of the most frequent barriers to care are network adequacy, prior authorizations (PAs) for things that did not need them previously, and the even greater challenges, such as linking

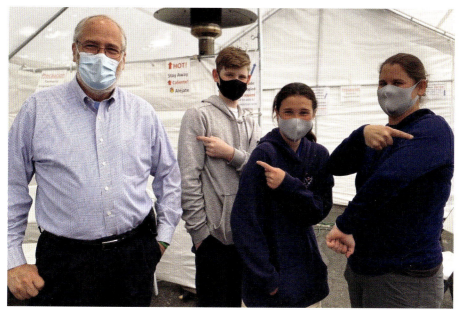

**Patients with Dr. David M. Millsaps, MD, FAAP, point to their vaccination sites.**

at-risk children to mental health assistance and children not receiving medications at the pharmacy of choice for the families.

**Some successes:**

- Single preferred drug list that all plans must follow
- Single credentialing process
- Newborn care protected for ninety days after birth (any Medicaid enrolled doctor will be paid in-network rate by any plan, even if the doctor is out-of-network)
- Existing prior authorizations (PAs) stand for 60 days post-launch
- Care covered at in-network rates for any providers
- Improvement to auto-assignment problems/catching a flawed auto-assignment algorithm for one plan
- Foster Care Plan delayed until 2023 (Yet another statewide plan to be implemented when the shock to the system that occurred when NC expanded from one Medicaid payor to six payors eventually abates.)
- Panel changes
- EPSDT protected in "pay and chase" when Medicaid-eligible patients covered under a parent's private insurance
- More claims testing than originally planned by the PHPs prior to going live
- New codes must be paid in forty-five days of notification or PHPs pay penalties
- Troubleshooting for beneficiaries

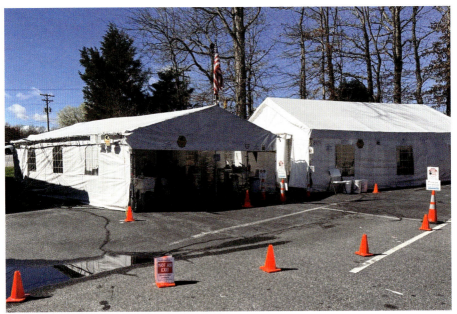

**COVID-19 Incident Command Center**

- AmeriHealth and WellCare ended copays for Medicaid visits for kids (programming error; feds prohibit Medicaid copays for kids)
- Seem to be getting close on a form to switch primary care provider (PCP) that can be signed while in the provider's office
- Original Medicaid transformation "guardrail provisions" on prior authorizations and payment at in-network rates extended

The pandemic brought challenges and uncharted territory for physicians in all specialities. The practical and often simple, common-sense recommendations by pediatricians put NCPeds in a leadership role as we confronted and adapted to the unexpected circumstances of a global medical and humanitarian crisis.

## Practice Support and Innovation During the COVID-19 Pandemic

by Susan Huffman, CMPE, and David Millsaps, MD, FAAP

The NC Pediatric Society leadership faced the COVID-19 virus, and quickly mobilized a virtual lifeboat of support for physicians and practice administrators through weekly "Solution Share" meetings and guidance to a host of resources.

Solution Share is the title given to the 5:30 p.m. Zoom sessions the leadership began convening in Spring 2020, early in the pandemic. The executive director provides the technology and funds the Zoom contract, and the president helps the executive director facilitate discussion that lasts no longer than thirty minutes. Participants usually include thirty to forty pediatricians, practice administrators, allied health professionals, and other child advocacy partners of the society. Sometimes, guest speakers from state government or academic medicine make brief presentations and conduct question-and-answer discussions. Most participants have found these conversations quite valuable as they chart their courses through the unknown waters of COVID-19.

Solution Share provided a forum for the membership to actively brainstorm with others and share ideas and solutions to the common problems all practices faced: PPE shortages: COVID-19 testing and time frame for results; parking lot and virtual check-ins and work-ups; telehealth; infection control; masking for patients and staff; air purification; change in the office pathway for sick and well patients; COVID-19 vaccinations; available grants; insurance coding; and, not the least of all, keeping practitioners and staff well and the practices financially solvent.

> The NC Pediatric Society leadership faced the COVID-19 virus, and quickly mobilized a virtual lifeboat of support for physicians and practice administrators.

In early 2020, as COVID-19 was making its entrance into the United States, Unifour Pediatrics personnel stopped to consider the "what-ifs" of what was surely about to arrive! The first thought was to try to keep patients and families safe by placing those who displayed COVID-19 symptoms (or had experienced possible exposure to the virus) in an open-air environment to reduce virus transmission.

I turned to my past wilderness medicine search and rescue experience in setting up Incident Command Centers, providing improvised rapid response coordinating logistics, infrastructure, and control services. In early March 2020, we quickly constructed outdoor walled canopies to triage and treat potentially infectious patients. The parking lot structure quickly evolved into a 1,200-square-foot clerical and clinical setting complete with power; sink and hygiene facilities; telephones; laptops and printers with Wi-Fi access and network switches; air conditioning; fans; heaters; patient check-in area; lab machines; twelve parent/child clinical treatment areas; and entrance into two private exam modules. This setup is much too elaborate to call it merely a tent!

At every level, the COVID-19 virus caused the practice of medicine to adapt with the changing environment. Elizabeth Hudgins, executive director of NCPeds, worked diligently to send detailed weekly updates across the state. With her "Weekly Wrap," she kept practices updated with the changing Medicaid guidelines and coding to assist practices, and conveniently provided links to join the multiple weekly webinars as practices worked out the new choreography of patient care.

Shelter-in-place orders and virus quarantine guidelines impacted patient visit numbers, and, as a result, practices experienced drastic declines in revenue. NCPeds leadership met with Medicaid representatives to communicate the fragile condition of outpatient front-line patient care. Through their advocacy, Medicaid broadened telehealth coding and reimbursement guidelines, and provided financial relief through a lengthened period of increased fees and doubling of the Per-Member Per-Month (PMPM) care management payment provided to practices under the Community Care of NC Medicaid Managed Care protocols.

In every region, childhood vaccination rates started to decline. Practices found innovative ways to reassure families with increased disinfection practices, temperature checks, changes of office hours, creation of special blocks of appointment times when no sick children could be admitted to offices, and dedicated staff members to supervise well-child appointments. These protected environments enabled well visits to surge and stabilize not only the immunization health of patients, but the financial viability of practices.

Social media, practice websites, and patient portals became even more valuable as communication tools to show parents our new contactless check in and practice procedures. Aerial videos demonstrated the route through the parking lot and the step-by-step office visit procedures.

Parents were very receptive to the "waiting room" and the patient "work up" now being completed in the comfort of their motor vehicles, and in the children's familiar environments with their toys and snacks. Many types of patient visit work ups can be completed prior to their appointments, thereby reducing waiting time and increasing efficiency.

Leaders of NCPeds, the NCPeds Solution Share, and the weekly newsletter resources provided immeasurable support as we planned and implemented safe care for patients. The ideas shared by physicians and managers helped us all. We clung together and survived! Thanks to NCPeds for providing the lifeboat!

# NCPeds Support for Pediatricians in Independent Practice

**by Lourdes Pereda, MD, FAAP**

My involvement with the NC Pediatric Society (NCPeds) started during my first Open Forum meeting after I moved to North Carolina in 2004. This was the first meeting I attended where pediatricians were welcoming, and I could feel the Southern hospitality right from the beginning, especially during the individual introductory greetings. I could feel the difference after working in two other states.

As a new pediatrician, NCPeds helped me understand state Medicaid and insurance programs. The leadership deals with them as a group, helping all the members when problems arise. Not only do they help the members, but they also help nonmembers by resolving practice financial problems.

During one of these meetings, I talked with a dear friend who was selling her practice. She encouraged me to open my own practice, and gave me helpful tips on starting from scratch. I also bought some of her medical equipment and furniture for my new practice.

One of the benefits of NCPeds is their networking with other state and national medical organizations. Leaders with NCPeds recommended that I attend the Leadership College of the NC Medical Society, which was a year-long learning experience with incredible instructors and research opportunities. It concluded with presentations to the leadership group concerning our research in our communities. They taught us how to create bridges in our communities to work with like-minded organizations to improve the health and well-being of our population.

NCPeds also sponsored me to attend the AAP National Advocacy Conference in Washington, DC. This is possible for any member interested in advocacy. This experience was eye-opening and helped me understand that not all progressive changes can be accomplished from inside our communities. Some require action by government leaders, especially legislators. Pediatricians from the fifty states and Puerto Rico visited Capitol Hill, and we met with senators and representatives of our own states, explained to them our problems, and suggested possible solutions, always advocating for our patients. It was an intense and busy meeting, but very interesting. I have returned to this meeting as often as possible to be up to date on state and national child advocacy issues.

During one of these meetings, I met Julie Linton, MD, FAAP, a passionate advocate and leader of AAP initiatives on immigrant health. When she was a faculty member at Wake Forest University School of medicine, she created the NCPeds Immigration

Task Force. She invited me to join this group, and we authored papers published in medical journals.

My journey with NCPeds has brought me many rewards, the latest one being invited to become a board member of this amazing organization. I am very thankful and grateful for what they do on behalf of our children, families, and pediatricians in North Carolina.

## Overcoming Rural Health Challenges

by Joey Bell, MD, FAAP (Lumbee)

Because I was born and raised in Pembroke, coming back home to practice medicine after residency was an easy decision. I thought that I was prepared for the challenges of practicing in rural southeastern North Carolina, but I was overwhelmed by the barriers embedded in the culture: poverty (our practice was about 80 percent Medicaid), illiteracy (more than 80 percent of third graders were not reading at grade level), and the lack of pediatric specialties available because the University of North Carolina and Duke University are a three hour drive away. This high demand for health care taxed the mind, body, and spirit. Despite the aforementioned challenges, the one thing that struck me the most was the lack of a voice these children had at the state level . . . especially the Native American children. I felt that there had to be a way to level the playing field for the children in the region. Enter the NCPeds!

After some discussion with my colleagues, I felt encouraged to become a member of NCPeds. It seemed as if they were working on many of the challenges that kept me awake at night—especially Medicaid payment and special programs for at-risk children. Their advocacy efforts, including lobbying the legislature, were making and continue to make great strides for children. I have served on the executive committee of NCPeds and the American Academy of Pediatrics' Committee on Native American Child Health, not only to give support for the children of southeastern North Carolina but to bring attention to the unique health care needs of all Native American children.

Through their advocacy efforts, NCPeds has achieved numerous wins for the children: a great immunization rate, NC Health Choice (our CHIP program), and a free vaccine program for our uninsured/Medicaid low-income patients are just a few of the countless advocacy efforts spearheaded by NCPeds.

*Editor's Note: Between 1965—when Congress created Medicaid—and today, NCPed's leadership and infrastructure have given practicing pediatricians, general and academic, opportunities to work with state government administrators and elected officials to assure that ALL North Carolina pediatricians can afford to offer comprehensive health services to ALL children who present needing health services. Joey Bell, MD, FAAP, is just one example of a pediatrician who chose to practice in his very impoverished home county and was able to afford to do this because of the efforts of NCPeds.*

## Supporting The Rural Solo Pediatrician In Practice

**by Beverly Edwards, MD, FAAP**

I know my small, rural, eastern North Carolina practice would not exist if it were not for NCPeds.

I grew up in Raleigh and attended East Carolina University School of Medicine. I met many great pediatricians there and heard about many more who were active in child advocacy. In eastern North Carolina, Dr. Dave Tayloe Sr.'s name was well known, as Dr. Dave Tayloe Jr.'s. is too, for the generous time and attention they have given to those of us who need NCPeds. I first joined NCPeds in the late 1990s, just before my first Board of Pediatrics Recertification Exam. I needed a village to learn and review, and I found that community with NCPeds. I am quite shy, but everyone I met was friendly and helpful. I passed the exam and made sure I became active in NCPeds, at least during recent years. The meetings were enjoyable and, believe it or not, I saw both Asheville and Myrtle Beach for the first time at NCPeds meetings.

During the last decade, NCPeds has been a critical advocate for me as the Affordable Care Act rollout began, causing great disruption within the business efficiency of my practice. I was on the verge of financial collapse when Drs. Christoph Diasio and Graham Barden, co-chairs of the NCPeds Pediatric Council, took my case zealously, and weekly, to the powers that be in Raleigh until our practice was up to speed and flourishing. I can never thank them enough.

I have learned a lot about child advocacy from Dr. Kathleen Clarke-Pearson, whom I met at an NCPeds meeting. Dr. Clarke-Pearson convinced NCPeds to pay my expenses so I could attend the 2018 National Legislative Conference, where gun control legislation was the focus. My children have friends who have been killed or wounded by gun violence. It is a blight that affects all of us, not just our children.

Lastly, I make it a point to meet the officers of NCPeds. They find it in themselves to make time to keep all members educated, represent NCPeds in multiple venues, and take care of their own patients and families as well. I admire them and am grateful for all the well-planned meetings, the daily information we receive, and the sense of community I feel when gathered in-person or by Zoom.

# A Pediatrician in the North Carolina Legislature

by William R. Purcell, MD, FAAP

I was fortunate to have an opportunity to serve in the NC Senate for fifteen-and-a-half years beginning in 1997. For most of those years, I served as chair or co-chair of the Senate Health Care Committee. This gave me an opportunity to work closely with a number of health-related organizations: North Carolina Pediatric Society; North Carolina Medical Society; North Carolina Nurses Association; North Carolina Hospital Association; many medical specialty organizations; American Heart Association; American Cancer Society; Heart Disease and Stroke Prevention Task Force; NC Alliance for Health; NC Child Fatality Task Force; and several pharmaceutical companies.

None of these contacts were more important or more helpful than NCPeds. The help of NCPeds was needed, not only in deciding what issues were most important for North Carolina's children and their health care providers, but which issues should have priority as the NCPeds Health Care Committee developed its agendas.

Steve Shore, executive director of NCPeds, and John Rusher, the chapter legislative liaison, were always at health care committee meetings, and were frequently in my office with suggestions, advice, and consultation. I often heard from, and consulted with, many leaders of NCPeds, including Dr. Dave Tayloe Jr., Dr. Bob Schwartz, and many others. These individuals and fellow pediatricians across the state made important contacts with other legislators to ensure support of child health legislation as it moved through the legislative process.

I believe that working with the guidance and support of NCPeds makes it much easier for an individual pediatrician to have his or her particular practice issues properly presented and heard in the appropriate legislative committee.

With help from NCPeds and other organizations, we advanced a number of bills that could impact the health and well-being of North Carolina's children. A few of them are listed here:
- statewide standard for vending machine products sold during the school day
- statewide nutrition standards for school meals and after school snacks
- seat belt use enhancement requiring all passengers in a motor vehicle in forward motion to wear a seat belt
- all terrain vehicle regulations
- funds for defibrillators in public buildings
- an act to phase out the county share of the non-federal share of Medicaid costs
- animal exhibition (petting zoo) sanitation law – "Aedins law"

- bills banning smoking in public schools, public buildings, university campuses and especially in bars and restaurants
- prohibition of medicine administration in child care centers without the guardian's written permission – "Kaitlyn's law"
- act appropriating funds for the NC Aids Drug Assistance Program

And the list could go on.

During my more than fifteen years in the NC Senate, NCPeds and North Carolina's pediatricians were always present when needed. They provided essential support for the passage of the above listed bills, as well as other legislation and policies that affected children and their providers.

### Addendum: A Message to fellow pediatricians

*If there is interest in serving in the NC General Assembly, and if one is able, then I would without hesitation say, "go for it"! It can be a very challenging and rewarding experience with a wonderful opportunity to influence the health and well-being of children, often in a much broader way than one can in practice.*

# Advocating for Children Over the Years

**by Chuck Willson, MD, FAAP**

As a pediatrician, job one was seeing my patients in the office when they needed care. Often, after caring for their immediate needs, the ultimate outcome of my care was dependent on societal factors at the family level, the community level, the state level, and the national level.

The open forum of NCPeds gives concerned pediatricians the infrastructure support they need to address the "outside the practice" factors that impact child health and outcomes.

For a while in the 1980s, we could not purchase DPT vaccines due to lawsuits such as the one that Dave Tayloe Jr.'s father (see *Big Dave: Visionary Leader*) suffered, driving up the cost of the vaccine. On a positive note, we all benefited when the Clinton administration enacted insurance coverage for low-income working families, the State Children's Health Insurance Program (SCHIP). When commercial Health Maintenance Organizations threatened to take over NC Medicaid, physician leaders came together to create Carolina Access and expanded it into the statewide Community Care of North Carolina (CCNC) partnership with Medicaid. In each of these instances, pediatricians advocating for children helped shape the outcomes.

Vaccine liability legislation, the CHIP bill, and organized support and defense of Carolina Access were only possible because of NCPeds' infrastructure and leadership.

Of course, the best advocates for children are the parents themselves. However, the parents often do not have the knowledge, time, or skill to advocate where and when decisions are being made. That is where pediatricians come in. We know our communities, our state, and even our nation. Working with medical professional organizations such as NCPeds, the American Academy of Pediatrics, the North Carolina Medical Society (NCMS) and the American Medical Association (AMA), we can provide societal leaders and legislators with the information they need to create better programs to support children and families.

While I was incredibly busy seeing patients, I enjoyed my work with these professional societies because there I could meet the extraordinary physicians who were doing the advocacy that was making a difference in children's lives. These physicians were and are my heroes.

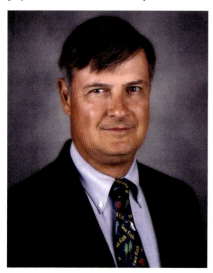

Chuck Willson, MD, FAAP

The NCPeds Open Forum was the foundation of our advocacy efforts throughout the years. When his father was wrongly accused of medical malpractice, Dave Tayloe Jr. led the effort to create the NC Childhood Vaccine Injury Compensation Program that made vaccines more available and affordable in NC. The program may have served as a model for national legislation. When my state senator held a news conference in Raleigh about the vaccine bill, he asked me, as the pediatrician for his family, to attend that news conference. Community relationships are powerful.

NCPeds provided the lobbyist, the public relations firm, and the key contact legislative network that enabled Dr. Dave Tayloe Jr. to assure passage of legislation to establish the NC Childhood Vaccine Injury Compensation Program.

Another great pediatric leader is David Bruton MD, from Southern Pines. He became friends with Governor Jim Hunt. Governor Hunt appointed him first to the state board of education, and later, he named David the secretary of NC Health and Human Services (NC DHHS). From that platform, Dr. Bruton and James Bernstein, the father of rural health in our country, designed a partnership between primary care physicians in our state with our state Medicaid program called Carolina Access, a medical home model. He also led the implementation of the Child Health Insurance Program (CHIP), called NC Health Choice.

Dr. Bruton needed the grassroots support of NCPeds membership to assure almost universal participation by physicians in Carolina Access, to defend Carolina Access from takeover by a hospital consortium, and to help key pediatricians and advocates work skillfully with a Democrat-controlled Senate and Republican-controlled House to pass model CHIP legislation.

Carolina Access started as nine pilot projects across NC that expanded statewide and became Community Care of North Carolina. One of those pilots was in my hometown, Greenville. We started with 12,500 Medicaid patients in Pitt County and eventually expanded the Community Care Plan of Eastern Carolina to over twenty counties with 140,000 patients. Children in these counties had enhanced access to primary care medical homes. Immunization rates soared and unnecessary use of the hospital emergency department plummeted. The state saved precious dollars. A state audit by Milliman (formerly Milliman and Robertson) estimated that Community Care of North Carolina saved NC Medicaid $950 million dollars during a five-year period. I was proud to serve as the medical director of our network, Community Care Plan of Eastern Carolina, for twelve years.

The open forum meetings served as the opportunity for bringing together administrators and physicians critical to the success of Carolina Access. With the

> Vaccine liability legislation, the CHIP bill, and organized support and defense of Carolina Access were only possible because of the infrastructure and leadership of NCPeds.

advocacy skills I learned in our NCPeds Open Forum, I became an emerging leader in the North Carolina Medical Society. I was nominated to the North Carolina Health and Wellness Trust Fund Commission. This Commission was funded by dollars received from the national tobacco settlement of 1998. We focused on improving the health of all North Carolinians by decreasing the numbers of children who started smoking, and we provided educational resources for physicians to help patients who were smokers to quit smoking. We had Tobacco Reality Unfiltered (TRU) chapters started in many high schools. Powerful, realistic statewide TV advertisements showed young adults suffering the consequences of years of smoking. We documented a decrease in the number of middle school children taking up tobacco use. Living in a county dependent on tobacco dollars, my leadership of this effort was not always comfortable; my next-door neighbor is a tobacco farmer.

Pediatrician advocates need coworkers who understand the importance of "outside the practice" advocacy work to improve the health and well-being of children and families, and to assure that all children have access to comprehensive health services in a medical home. Dr. Dave Tayloe Jr. has had practice partners who have allowed him to be away from the practice to lead "outside the practice" advocacy initiatives.

These "outside the practice" activities eventually took a toll on job one. I often had Community Care of Pitt County (CCP) meetings at 7 a.m. and arrived for hospital rounds late. Days off were spent on the road to Raleigh, Greensboro, and Asheville. While I loved what I was doing, my partners felt that I was not pulling my load in the practice. They asked me to cut back. I could not. I decided to take an offer to join the faculty of the Brody School of Medicine at East Carolina University (ECU) where I would have 50 percent of my time to work on advocacy and the other 50 percent would be practicing my first love, clinical pediatrics.

In the twilight of my career, I have learned how to better care for children with special health care needs, including those with developmental disabilities like autism. With all our education and experience, we pediatricians should make job one caring and advocating for these special children. We can have non-physician practitioners do the more routine care under our guidance. My mentor for this work is Olson Huff, MD, FAAP, a past president of NCPeds who started the NC Early Childhood Foundation to educate communities, schools, and political leaders about how to provide a positive environment for early brain growth and development. He established a center, now called the Olson Huff Center for Child Development, in Asheville. At the ECU medical school, I have learned another type of advocacy: teaching the next generation of pediatricians. Of all the jobs I do at ECU, I love teaching medical students and residents the most. After nineteen years in a busy pediatric practice, seeing forty to sixty patients a day, I felt that I had the necessary experience to teach outpatient pediatrics.

Mentorship is so important to the success of the profession of pediatrics. NCPeds has welcomed students and residents, creating special opportunities for these groups to participate in meetings of the chapter as members of the larger group and in small-group meetings designed to allow them to accomplish their short- and long-term goals.

Joining the medical school faculty also gave me the time to serve on the NC Medical Society's delegation to the American Medical Association (AMA). For twenty-two years, I went to meetings of the AMA House of Delegates twice a year. Bob Seligson, chief executive officer of NCMS, helped me win a spot on the AMA Council on Medical Service where I was able to advocate for a better health care system for all Americans. While not welcomed by all delegates, the council on medical service recommended that AMA support the Patient Protection and Affordable Care Act

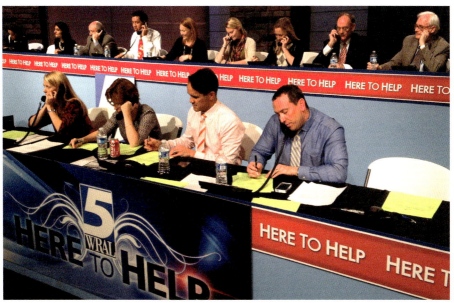

**NCPeds members participated in two WRAL Doctors on Call episodes.**

(Obamacare). After a heated discussion, the AMA House of Delegates agreed as policy that AMA would support the Affordable Care Act. Several members of the NC delegation resigned in protest. My firm belief is that until America has a high quality, affordable health care system for all Americans, our country will be vulnerable to threats such as COVID-19 and lifestyle induced morbidities and mortality.

Through the open forum, NCPeds has worked with state government leaders and administrators to assure that more than 90 percent of children have Medicaid, CHIP, or private health insurance. Pediatricians have played a vital role in convincing state medical societies and the AMA to work for federal and state reforms to increase the number of adults who have access to insurance that provides first-dollar coverage for preventive health services, affordable sick-care insurance, and fair payment for physicians—the three pillars of the child health insurance program in North Carolina.

As I worked with the NCPeds Executive Committee, I was elected to serve on the national nominating committee of the American Academy of Pediatrics. There, I was able to advocate for Dave Tayloe Jr's nomination to run for president of the academy. He won! So, Dave has been able to advocate for children at the community level, the state level, the national level, and the international level.

I must warn my colleagues that advocating for children is infectious. As your advocacy becomes recognized, you will be invited to more and more activities where your knowledge, skills, and experience are needed. Do not try to do it all. Another physician mentor, Walter Pories, MD, FACS, the first chair of surgery at the Brody School of Medicine once told me, "Chuck, I appreciate all your advocacy work, but you cannot do it all. I am the chair of our local museum of art. Because I am doing that, you do not need to."

We must teach other pediatricians in our communities to get involved in facets of advocacy that inspire them most. I am blessed that my wife, Wendy, has allowed me to serve children in these many ways because all of this advocacy work often takes me away from my home and family—although she has enjoyed the five AMA meetings in Honolulu! At an NCPeds meeting where I was handing over the presidency of that group to my successor, someone asked my oldest daughter, Ellen, if she felt that I had been neglecting her and her sisters by being away so much. Her response still brings tears to my eyes, "No, that's who he is." Now as a pediatric nurse, she even better understands the need for advocacy for children! Another daughter is a psychiatric nurse practitioner, and our third daughter is a veterinarian. They are all superb health care professionals, and each has taken up advocating for their patients. I am so proud!

> When it comes to doing our best for children every day, both as pediatricians and public advocates, well, sure! Why not?

I am so blessed to have chosen pediatrics as my career. To have parents ask me to care for their child is such a high honor!

## Pediatricians as Advocates? Why Not?

by David Hill, MD, FAAP

The sneaky thing about pediatricians is their calming voices. They can say the most alarming things, but with that voice you just don't notice. And no pediatrician has mastered this trick better than former NCPeds president, Dr. Peter Morris, perhaps because he's also an ordained minister.

So, when Peter dialed me up out of the blue sometime in 2009 and asked me to speak to a town hall meeting in the military bastion of Fayetteville, NC, in support of the "Obamacare" Affordable Care Act, I agreed with the equanimity of Daniel pausing to rest in the lion's den. "Sure," I said. "Why not?"

It was not until I arrived at the meeting and saw sheriff's deputies lining the walls that I wondered if I might be in just a bit over my head. Of course, I have cultivated my own version of this voice. I'm no Peter Morris, but I brought all the toddler-soothing mellifluousness I could muster to the restless crowd and barely shrank back from the podium when the yelling started, and the deputies stepped a few paces closer to the podium.

I'm not sure how I did, but Peter seemed happy, and soon thereafter another past president, Dr. Herb Clegg, called and, in his own melodious tones, suggested that I might serve on the NCPeds Executive Committee. "Sure," I said. "Why not?"

I suppose it was at one of those meetings where Dr. Kathleen Clarke-Pearson sidled up and, in the most calming imaginable way, asked if I might be interested in running for an open position on the executive committee of the AAP Council on Communications and Media (COCM), open because she was rotating off. "Sure," I said. "Why not?"

Shortly after I arrived, the COCM chair, Dr. Deborah Mulligan, suggested gently that I might take on the role of education chair, a role for which I had no discernable qualifications. "Sure," I said. "Why not?"

A couple of years later, AAP Executive Vice President Mark Del Monte grabbed my elbow and asked if I might succeed Deb as chair. "Sure," I said. "Why not?"

From there, it was on to the AAP Council Management Committee and, later this year, the chair position of that committee. Oh, and the Pediatrics on Call podcast. And editing Caring for Your Baby and Young Child: Birth to Age 5. And editing AAP pediatric patient education. Because . . . well, you know.

At every step of the way, my incredible colleagues at NCPeds have advised, supported, and bolstered me. I even have the honor of working beside another former NCPeds and AAP President, Dr. Dave Tayloe Jr. He continues to inspire me in my mission daily, and his voice grounds me when the challenges of pediatric practice and advocacy feel overwhelming. Because when it comes to doing our best for children every day, both as pediatricians and public advocates, well, sure! Why not?

# Part VI

## Reflections of Friends and Partners in Advocacy

# Impact on Child Health Outcomes
# at a Population Level

by Thomas F. Boat, MD, FAAP

I arrived in Chapel Hill as chair of the UNC Department of Pediatrics in June 1982. I was quickly informed that I would be attending the fall meeting of NCPeds in Pinehurst and that this was mandatory, because academic and community-based pediatricians worked closely together in that venue. This was a new experience for me as my previous contact with state pediatric societies in Minnesota and Ohio suggested little interest on the part of most faculty in academic centers. Little did I know how this partnership, among other factors, had advanced the society in North Carolina to a level of energy and accomplishment that was likely unexcelled at that time and that has kept NCPeds at the forefront of state pediatric organizations.

At the first meeting, chaired by "Big Dave" Tayloe from little Washington, it was quickly apparent that NCPed's goals were advocacy oriented, focusing not only on clinical practice enhancement, but access to full medical surveillance and care for all children in the state. I was amazed that the assembly was connected through individuals to important decision makers in the state health department, the governor's office, and the legislative assemblies. Not only that, but they were seriously discussing the hiring of a lobbyist in Raleigh to facilitate and build on those connections, a plan that was implemented in the next year. NCPeds clearly had laid an admirable foundation for continuing progress.

What NCPeds was able to do in the next forty years has been equally amazing: better coverage for Medicaid qualified children, better reimbursement for physician participation in Medicaid, universal Early and Periodic Screening, Diagnostic and Treatment (EPSDT) screening for young children, and the adoption of other programs of importance to children and families of NC. Added to the statewide effort has been very successful partnerships of pediatricians with their communities, including local government, schools, and health systems to improve not only physical but social-emotional health and well-being, particularly of disadvantaged children. NCPeds opened its doors to non-physician members such as practice managers and has grown remarkably. Participation, I am sure, has been aided by the admirable inclusivity of the society, an example being attendance by state level health management officials at the meetings. Another lesson to be learned from the North Carolina experience is that sustained advocacy efforts over years and decades do pay off.

North Carolina is now known throughout the national pediatric ranks as a place where children access health care and monitoring with a minimum of barriers.

North Carolina is now known throughout the national pediatric ranks as a place where children access health care and monitoring with a minimum of barriers.

In no small part, that can be attributed to the unwavering effort and notable effectiveness of NCPeds and its remarkable leadership. This book provides details concerning society achievements and provides a roadmap to successful efforts on the part of other states and regions. This book documents that individual and collective ingenuity, clear and collective purpose, strategic planning, and relentless plan implementation has worked to the advantage of children and families, an effort that can be modeled across the country.

*Fifty Years of Advocacy: The North Carolina Pediatric Society* is important reading for all child health providers, and particularly for all those who can and should impact child health outcomes at a population level.

## Front-Line Partners of the Secretary: Confronting the Pandemic with the NC Department of Health and Human Services

by Charlene Wong, MD, MSHP; Mandy Cohen, MD, MPH

In the work of the North Carolina Department of Health and Human Services (NC DHHS) to promote the health and well-being of children and families, North Carolina's pediatricians are our front-line partners. In this commentary, we describe the essential role that the North Carolina Pediatric Society (NCPeds) played in our response to the COVID-19 pandemic and look ahead to our continued partnership to support whole child and family health.

During the COVID-19 pandemic, the leadership, especially NCPeds President Christoph Diasio and Executive Director Elizabeth Hudgins and members of NCPeds, served in multiple roles that were critical in our response.

First, pediatricians and health care clinicians were consistently among the highest rated as trusted messengers in North Carolina in multiple rounds of market research conducted by NC DHHS. Pediatricians were the steady voice sought by parents and communities as we moved from promoting the three Ws (Wear a face mask.

Wash your hands. Watch your distance.) to encouraging COVID-19 vaccines for adults, teens, and children. In a time of such uncertainty for caregivers who were trying to make the right decisions for their children as usual routines were disrupted, pediatricians were the ones answering questions and guiding their patients through this challenging time. We called on NCPeds members multiple times to participate in fireside chats, cafecitos (discussions over coffee), and webinars so that families across the state could benefit from their expertise.

Second, pediatricians provided essential health care for children infected with or exposed to COVID-19. As COVID-19 guidelines and resources evolved, NCPeds collected, edited, and disseminated important clinical information about testing and treatment statewide in regular email communications and solution share Zoom discussions at 5:30 p.m. on Tuesdays.

Third, pediatricians continue to play a vital role in vaccinating children and their families against COVID-19. Here again, NCPeds was a leading voice in providing feedback to shape our vaccination efforts, always advocating for solutions that promote more equitable distribution of COVID-19 vaccines across ages. The role of pediatricians and NCPeds grew even more important as COVID-19 vaccines became available to younger children, and parents preferred for their children to be vaccinated in their primary care medical homes as opposed to at pharmacies or health department clinics. In addition, we are appreciative of pediatricians facilitating vaccinations not only for children but also offering primary series or booster vaccines to adult family members.

The impact of the COVID-19 pandemic on children has been profound, shining a spotlight on how we, as a state, need to strengthen the systems that support children and their families. Our department's vision for children and families is for children to be healthy and able to thrive in safe, stable, and nurturing families, schools, and communities. The health and well-being of children and families are a current top priority area for NC DHHS. In our 2021-23 strategic plan, building a strong infrastructure to increase access to child and family well-being services is a key objective. In 2022, we established a Division of Child and Family Well-Being that brings together complementary programs that support the health, social, and emotional needs of children, youth, and families in North Carolina.

Our ongoing work with NCPeds is a fundamental component of our child-and-family-focused efforts across the department. Prioritized areas as we move into COVID-19 recovery include child behavioral health, child welfare, food insecurity for children and families, and maternal and infant health. NCPeds has driven improvements in each of these areas. Examples include improving services for children cared for by the child welfare system through the Fostering Health program and promoting the needs of children, families, and their clinical providers when we have major shifts in our health care landscape, such as during the creation and implementation of Community Care of North Carolina and the ongoing Medicaid transformation process.

We could not be more grateful for the strength of our state's American Academy of Pediatrics chapter (NCPeds) and for the long partnership with NC DHHS.

# NCPeds' Friends in North Carolina State Government

by Gerri Mattson, MD, MSPH, FAAP; Kelly Kimple, MD, MPH, FAAP;
Betsey Cuervo Tilson, MD, MPH, FAAP; Shannon Dowler, MD, FAAFP

Much of the success of NCPeds in advocacy for the children, families, and pediatricians of our state is attributable to the progressive collaboration involving the physicians who work in state government and society leaders. Some of these state government administrators offer their comments below to bring the NCPeds–state government relationship to life.

> I credit NCPeds with feeling happy and hopeful, even in the midst of all that is going on for children, families, and providers in our state these days.

**GERRI MATTSON, MD, MSPH, FAAP, NC DEPARTMENT OF HEALTH AND HUMAN SERVICES**

NCPeds has given me so many professional and personal opportunities to build relationships, find mentors and mentees, and partner with amazing colleagues. I credit NCPeds with feeling happy and hopeful, even in the midst of all that is going on for children, families, and providers in our state these days. My passion has been to increase systems and processes that support family-centered whole child care, especially for children and youth with special health care needs and their families.

Many years ago, NCPeds provided my first home to find colleagues and work on this passion through the Committee on Children with Disabilities. I want to briefly highlight how NCPeds lifted up children in foster care as one example of their efforts to improve the health and well-being of Children and Youth with Special Health Care Needs (CYSHCN). Many years of meetings with NCPeds members and partners across the state led to the creation of Fostering Health NC. Fostering Health NC has improved the quality of care for children in foster care to meet American

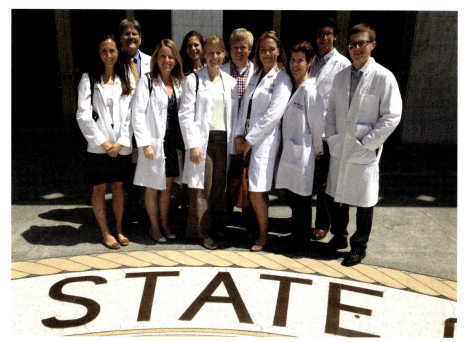

NCPeds members, residents, and medical students are frequent visitors to the NC General Assembly.

Academy of Pediatrics standards across the state. Fostering Health NC strengthened the coordination among families (foster and biological parents), DSS (Department of Social Services) case workers, medical homes, and care managers in more than half of our counties. Fostering Health NC is invaluable as staff and pediatricians continue to advocate for ongoing issues: processes to facilitate enrollment of foster children into Medicaid; important elements of the specialized plan for children in foster care; and the needs of youth formerly in foster care. Thank you to NCPeds for all that you do in partnership with us and so many others to improve the lives of CYSHCN and their families!

### KELLY KIMPLE, MD, MPH, FAAP, NC DEPARTMENT OF HEALTH AND HUMAN SERVICES

As a pediatrician and director of the NC Maternal and Child Health with the NC Department of Health and Human Services, I have witnessed NCPeds as a strong voice, a committed advocate, and an invaluable partner to serve children and families across North Carolina. They share perspectives, inform policy, provide expertise, improve processes, solve problems, and are that powerful, constant voice to improve systems that serve children. Whether it is the dedicated work to roll out COVID-19 vaccination of our state's children, with a focus on trusted medical homes, ensuring routine vaccination access, or helping address the many health issues that face children—adverse childhood experiences, obesity, mental health conditions, smoking and vaping, infant and childhood injury and death—NCPeds and NC DHHS are committed and eager to do it together. As we continue to work as partners for the health and well-being of individuals and the population, in pediatric form, I will "reach out and read" in Dr. Seuss' style:

> With NCPeds, I would want to be in our shoes.
> We can help families in so many ways that we choose.
> We create opportunities, tend our programs with care.
> About some you'll say, "I think this family should go there."
> With your head full of brains and your shoes full of feet,
> we want to send all families down the good street.
> There are so many ways to address these problems.
> And we all have the passion to get out and solve them.
> With immunizations, Fostering Health, breastfeeding and others . . .
>    we really are on a mission!
> Oh! The Places You'll Go
> So many needs in families that can't wait.
> We have a vision, a mission
> and we can be great!
> NCPeds will ride high!
> Ready for anything under the sky!
> Ready because
> you were born to fly!
> Oh, the places you'll go!
> You are off to great places!
> Today is your day!
> Your mountain is waiting.
> So . . . get on your way!

**BETSEY CUERVO TILSON, MD, MPH, FAAP**
**NC DEPARTMENT OF HEALTH AND HUMAN SERVICES**

I have provided pediatric primary care, served as a medical director for Community Care of North Carolina, and now I serve as the NC Department of Health and Human Services State Health Director and Chief Medical Officer. As a pediatrician involved in several major innovations and changes in North Carolina, and as a long-standing member of NCPeds, I have seen the power of advocacy and leadership of

NCPeds in shaping and improving the system of health for our children and families. NCPeds led and shaped Community Care of North Carolina, which wrapped population health strategies, care management, and systems of care around patients covered by Medicaid and enrolled in primary care medical homes. NCPeds was a powerful force in supporting and advocating for systematically addressing some fundamental social drivers of health, including food insecurity, housing deficiencies, and Adverse Childhood Experiences (ACEs). NCPeds was instrumental in helping guide the design of the transformation of our Medicaid program to Medicaid Managed Care in a way that served children and families. NCPeds was an invaluable partner in our state's response to the COVID-19 pandemic, and played a critical role in provider communication, giving input to policy changes, and facilitating access to testing, vaccine, and treatment. North Carolina, our families, and our children are better because of the tireless and dedicated work of NCPeds.

### SHANNON DOWLER, MD, FAAFP, CHIEF MEDICAL OFFICER FOR NC MEDICAID

As NC Medicaid Chief Medical Officer, when I think of the NC Pediatric Society (NCPeds), I immediately get reflux—like the kind of heartburn that has you reaching for a bottle of Tums! The truth is, that is a really good thing for the health of the state. I know when I get a phone call or a meeting request that something is happening that needs to be investigated. It is safe to say, "They keep us on our toes." NCPeds brings a number of assets to the table that I believe makes their impact so strong:

**They are persistent.** You cannot escape them. And just to be sure, they always keep a meeting on the books because something will invariably come up.

**They care—like, really, really care.** If we have a policy or procedure in place that is to the disadvantage of a Medicaid beneficiary, they are going to make sure we know it. If we initiated a process that disrupts the medical home or makes it harder for a pediatrician to do his or her job, they are going to make sure we know it and bring opportunities to us, including legislation.

**They are (almost always) right.** (I mean, no one is perfect, right?) The pediatric collective is incredibly knowledgeable about many facets of health care and in a breadth of areas: politics, practice management, systems of care. Before something is brought to our team, the homework has already been done and they are ready to define the problem and often bring a proposed solution or two.

**They are consistent.** While relative times of silence might be kind of nice (cough, cough), their leadership is constantly reaching out to practices to understand what is working and what is not working and bringing opportunities to us. They are generous with their praise and support of the work the team is doing, even when the outcome is not exactly how they would like it to be. If we agree to disagree, it is done amicably and respectfully.

**They are connected.** When we solve problems and seek solutions together, I have no doubt their network is hard at work in the background communicating. Our communication is bidirectional as well. When the team is looking for consensus, expert input, or guidance on a policy, we can always lean on them to shake the bushes and bring a variety of superstars to the table.

While I occasionally grumble, I more often count on these persistent, caring, wise, consistent, and connected partners to help the team and me do the best we can for the health of the Medicaid population, their families, and the providers in NC.

## Collaboration with NC Child

by Michelle Hughes, MSW

As the former executive director of NC Child and a long-time child advocate in North Carolina, I have always been deeply grateful for the advocacy of NCPeds. Not only is NCPeds an incredibly active and effective voice for children, but their voice is grounded in science, balanced, and always focused on the well-being of children first. We worked on so many policy and systems issues together over the years that I cannot count them all—from childhood vaccines, Medicaid transformation, early childhood mental health, children with special health care needs, the health of children in foster care, and so much more!

Throughout my years at NC Child, I was always thankful for NCPeds' collaborative approach, expertise, indefatigable spirit, and ability to adapt in quickly changing times to focus on what would most benefit our most vulnerable children. I know without a doubt that NC Child's partnership with NCPeds strengthened our collective advocacy for children and families in our state, as the staff and leadership of NCPeds are some of the most powerful and passionate advocates for children in North Carolina.

## Collaboration with the NC Academy of Family Physicians

by Gregory K. Griggs, MPA, CAE

The North Carolina Academy of Family Physicians (NCAFP) and the NC Pediatric Society (NCPeds) have worked together for as long as anyone can remember. The two organizations have shared so many common advocacy goals that cooperation and collaboration are only natural.

When Steve Shore first served NCPeds as executive director, his office, for a time, was in the NCAFP headquarters. When I had the pleasure of taking over as the exec for NCAFP, Steve was there to help mentor me on my new journey. And I hope I returned the favor just a bit when Elizabeth Hudgins took over as executive director of NCPeds.

But the two organizations have been intertwined much more than just supporting each other's staff. We have shared many common goals and projects. For example, the two organizations were leaders in the "Into the Mouths of Babes" dental fluoride varnish program, collaborating with others on research, and then advocacy, to convince NC Medicaid to cover the service. North Carolina truly led the nation on this important service to improve the oral health of young children.

Over the years, the two organizations also have worked together with so many in state government including the NC Division of Public Health, NC Office of Rural Health, and NC Medicaid program. In fact, to this day, Elizabeth and I still meet monthly with the leadership of our state's Medicaid program, representing the needs of primary care.

**And when COVID-19 hit, who did I turn to for a partner? As usual, NCPeds.**

For years, we worked together with Community Care of NC (CCNC), striving to improve the care of our state's Medicaid recipients. We fought Medicaid managed care together until legislation became inevitable. Then, together, we turned our attention to making the move to managed care as successful as possible, working to minimize the impact on patients and physicians alike.

One of my great personal pleasures while at NCAFP was playing just a small part in the NCPeds lawsuit over administrative fees for vaccines. Sitting with Elizabeth and physician leaders from NCPeds in a Goldsboro courtroom to ensure our member physicians were getting paid appropriately for providing vaccines to our state's children was quite simply remarkable.

And when COVID-19 hit, who did I turn to for a partner? As usual, NCPeds. The two groups, along with NC Area Health Education Centers (NC AHEC), Community Care of NC (CCNC), and the NC Psychiatric Association, conducted a series of webinars to help our members navigate both the clinical and financial impacts of COVID-19. We advocated to get testing supplies, personal protective equipment, and, ultimately, vaccines into the hands of primary care physicians.

Whether it is behavioral health integration in primary care practices, access to care, vaccines, the pandemic, or protecting adolescent consent, NCPeds has always been a leading advocate for children and other patients of all ages. It truly has been a pleasure to work with the leadership of NCPeds throughout my seventeen-year tenure with the NC Academy of Family Physicians.

# Collaboration with the NC Psychiatric Association

by Robin Huffman

In some ways, psychiatry has always been "of two minds" in our advocacy work in North Carolina. We stand proudly with the house of medicine, even though more people than we like to admit are never quite clear if it is psychiatrists or psychologists who are physicians or medical doctors. That confusion is probably strengthened because much of the NC Psychiatric Association's (NCPA) presence and advocacy is in coalition with mental health professional organizations in our mutual work to ensure parity in insurance coverage and funding for adequate mental health and addiction services and infrastructure. But I have noticed that when I represent psychiatry at big meetings with all the medical subspecialties, who do I sit with? Pediatricians and Family Medicine. I don't think that is an accident.

Over the decades, psychiatry has found a strong advocacy partner with pediatricians and NCPeds. From my earliest days as executive director of the NC Psychiatric Association (NCPA), we were invited to committee meetings of NCPeds, chaired by the likes of Drs. Jane Foy and Marian Earls. Together we grappled with mental health access to care for kids and issues related to our public mental health system reform that continues today. I recall difficult discussions about the ethics of screening kids for mental health issues if it is impossible to get them quickly seen by psychiatrists or mental health professionals.

Since the early 2000s, NCPA has been on a quest with NCPeds—first with Steve Shore and now Elizabeth Hudgins—and with the NC Academy of Family Physicians to acknowledge whole-person care and recognize the importance of screening and treating mental disorders to improve the overall health of patients.

I recall a meeting, held in a small meeting room at Wake Forest in 2002, with Dr. Foy, Steve Shore, psychiatrist Dr. Art Kelley, and a few others where we discussed the possibilities of replicating the Massachusetts MCPAP model. In this program, psychiatrists were available for telephone consults with pediatric practices. Today that model operates here and is called the NC Psychiatry Access Line (NC-PAL).

In 2006, NCPA jumped on the opportunity when invited to become a partner in the ICARE partnership that sought to create "an Integrated, Collaborative, Accessible,

Through my almost quarter century of working with members and leadership of NCPeds, I continue to admire and be impressed by the strong advocacy of pediatricians for children and youth.

Respectful and Evidence-based health care system by encouraging cooperation among behavioral health and medical professionals across NC." Sitting at the table with NCPeds, the NC Academy of Family Physicians, Community Care of North Carolina (CCNC), and others was the beginning of a long and fruitful partnership.

Through the progressive joint efforts with ICARE and the advent of the Center of Excellence for Integrated Care, primary care and psychiatry achieved successes in reconnecting the head to the body. Collaborating with each other and CCNC, we were able to work with NC Medicaid to adopt codes for the Collaborative Care Model, which is a model that brings psychiatric consultation to pediatric and primary care practices.

The realities of a worldwide pandemic on private practice brought psychiatry and pediatrics even closer. Our weekly meetings to plan "Navigating COVID-19" webinars resulted in other, bigger-picture conversations of ways primary care and psychiatry could change the world. Who knew that the challenges of a worldwide pandemic would forge even stronger ties and provide a platform for making some of these whole-person-care ideas a reality?

Through my almost quarter century of working with members and leadership of NCPeds, I continue to admire and be impressed by the strong advocacy of pediatricians for children and youth. You are fierce and fearless advocates for children. Our state is a better place because of your work, and the North Carolina Psychiatric Association is honored to work with you.

## Solving Problems for North Carolina's Children

by Allen Dobson Jr., MD, FAAFP

My thirty-plus-year history working with the leadership of the NC Pediatric Society began when I was a young family physician practicing in Mt. Pleasant, North

Carolina, and a new leader in the North Carolina Academy of Family Physicians (NCAFP). Working in my community introduced me to the dedication of local pediatric leaders such as George Engstrom, Frank Niblock, Linny Baker, and John Benbow, with whom I had the privilege of working on a number of medical issues such as school nursing; improved ADHD screening, evaluation, and treatment; and improving access for Medicaid patients at the beginning of the Carolina Access program. It was this local physician leadership in our community that would enable it to become the home for one of the first networks for Carolina Access/Community Care networks of NC (CCNC).

My collaboration with NCPeds over the years has involved many issues and projects, but I want to highlight three that illustrate the principles that I believe to be drivers of their work and effectiveness.

When I was the President of NCAFP in 1998–99, we were summoned to a meeting, along with leaders of NCPeds, and Jim Bernstein, director of Medicaid and the Office of Rural Health. Dr. Jim Bawden, pediatric dentist and former dean of the School of Dentistry at UNC, presented to us the results of a pilot he had conducted with local pediatricians. His aim was to reduce the significant amount of operative dental disease in young children in North Carolina, particularly among Medicaid-insured children, by having primary care physicians provide improved dental screening, better oral health education of parents, and to apply fluoride varnish beginning at the eruption of the first tooth and continuing every three months through six treatments. His pilot showed significant positive results.

Medicaid was willing to pay for the services if we could train and convince pediatricians and family physicians to implement the services. We accepted the challenge and worked collaboratively with the NCPeds leadership to participate in the Continuing Medical Education (CME) activities and training necessary to implement the program statewide. The program, now known as "Into the Mouth of Babes," became a national model. NCPeds values collaboration and innovation! (see *Into the Mouths of Babes*)

In 2005, I had the privilege of succeeding Jim Bernstein as assistant secretary of health for the NC Department of Health and Human Services (DHHS) and becoming the Medicaid director in the second term of Governor Mike Easley. When Secretary Carmen Hooker Odom approached me about taking on the Medicaid director job in addition to assistant secretary, I was hesitant, but she allowed me to have a chief operating officer, Mark Benton, and much latitude in updating the operating structure of Medicaid. I am still thankful for the amazing team we had at Medicaid in those days. As with any such position, there are things you want to accomplish during your service to the state, but also you just keep your fingers crossed that some crisis does not sidetrack you.

My first major crisis occurred not a week after I officially started the job. It was legislative budget time, and the legislature was close to a final budget. Mark Benton, with our finance and budget staff, came to me to report that there had been an error made in our NC Health Choice (CHIP) budget projections. There was a decimal point error resulting in severe underreporting of the amount of funding needed for the next budget.

My trip to the NC General Assembly to report the error was not a pleasant one! The amount of funding would not cover the number of children currently enrolled. Because there were no additional state funds available late in the budget cycle, the result would be removing thousands of children from the NC Health Choice insurance program. I asked legislative leaders for a week to figure out options. I called NCPeds and NCAFP leaders to attend an emergency meeting, and their solution was that physicians would take a voluntary fee decrease to create the funding needed to keep the kids enrolled in the program, in exchange for placing the NC Health Choice kids into the CCNC program. Providers would receive a per-member-per-month (PMPM) primary care fee to soften the fee decrease, as well as a network PMPM fee to support care management and support services. CCNC was to get data from BCBS (Blue Cross and Blue Shield), who administered the NC Health Choice program at the time. This agreement kept thousands of children insured, and improved their care since they would be managed according to well-proven and successful CCNC program standards. NCPeds always puts children first!

I have had the privilege of working side-by-side with the amazing leaders of NCPeds over twenty years of developing CCNC into a national model of care. At every step of the way, pediatricians were in leadership roles, making access and quality of care better for North Carolinians of all ages. I am sure I will omit names and initiatives, but I must call out some of the most significant that come to mind. Our goal in further developing the Carolina Access program into CCNC was to do more than just give Medicaid patients better access to care, but also to improve care in the community by providing those who care for patients the resources they needed. When we developed Access II and III (now CCNC) as pilots, we experimented with several models. One was a statewide network of mainly pediatric practices. Drs. Steve Wegner, Dave Tayloe, and Joe Ponzi headed this network with assistance from other dedicated physicians. Steve Wegner became one of my closest colleagues and a major leader in the CCNC movement.

Over the years, the Access Care network, and Dr. Steve Wegner in particular, were leaders in not only many pediatric initiatives but also other projects such as establishing CCNC as a central support organization, obtaining and assisting with major Centers for Medicare and Medicaid (CMS) grants, and even running a nursing home polypharmacy pilot. Drs. Chuck Willson and Tom Irons collaborated with

Drs. John Benbow, George Engstrom, Linny Baker, and me in developing the community-based network that included Pitt and Cabarrus counties, and later became a major network model for CCNC. CCNC proved that organizing primary care physicians and giving them resources (care management and data) along with local collaboration with hospitals, health departments and other health care providers, significantly improved quality but also saved money. These principles were proven effective by repeated external evaluations of the program.

I had the pleasure of working directly with so many amazing pediatric leaders over the years, including David Bruton, who served as DHHS Secretary and can be credited with advancing Carolina Access and CCNC; Olson Huff; Marian Earls; Dennis Clements; Bill Stewart; Christoph Diasio; Jane Foy; and Susan Mims; to name just a few. NCPeds has provided continuous and ongoing leadership to NC.

It has been my pleasure to serve alongside some amazing colleagues and leaders, and I congratulate NCPeds for being an example to others nationally.

# Medicaid Advocacy Notes

by William Lawrence Jr., MD, FAAP

As a bright-eyed, bushy-tailed, former pediatric chief resident entering my first year of community pediatric practice, I had no idea what advocacy and the North Carolina Pediatric Society would ultimately mean for my career. Yet the seeds were firmly planted in medical school through the mentorship of Drs. Mike Lawless, Jane Foy, and Jimmy Simon, as well as through my mentors in residency, Drs. Joseph Wright and Tina Cheng. When I entered practice, Dr. Charlie Kennedy was my role model. My first experience with a Medicaid administrator occurred when I encountered a new patient with nutritional rickets who needed coverage for an over-the-counter vitamin; it was not the most pleasant conversation. But it did reveal to me the importance of understanding health policies and processes, and not just the clinical care of children. My first year of practice also coincided with the year in which expansion of the NC Community Access Program reached essentially statewide status. My practice experiences sprouted an interest in, and commitment to, understanding the Safety Net for children with Medicaid as a key component.

Seven years later, I was blessed with the opportunity to join the NC Division of Medical Assistance. It was a time in which the innovations of successive NC DHHS Secretaries David Bruton and Carmen Hooker-Odom were thriving. Community Care of NC had evolved, and was successfully expanding throughout all of the state and demonstrating nationally recognized impact. I was embraced by the leadership of NCPeds and fortunate to work collaboratively on a number of critical issues for

# NCPeds has provided a developing ground support system and source of resolve for all aspects of my personal and professional advocacy for children.

the Medicaid and NC Health Choice (CHIP) populations: quality improvement in asthma management; improving payment for vaccine administration; expanding access to nutritional counseling; and partnering with the dental community to improve access, as examples. We collaboratively sought and achieved a Medicaid transformation grant supporting establishment of the Perinatal Quality Collaborative of NC (PQCNC). NCPeds membership contributed significantly to the modernization of Medicaid clinical policies through participation in the NC Physician Advisory Group.

As an official of the Medicaid administration, touting the depth and effectiveness of the public-private partnerships that flourished in North Carolina to colleagues nationally always energized me. Needless to say, throughout my tenure in several leadership roles at the NC Division of Medical Assistance and beyond, NCPeds has provided a developing ground support system and source of resolve for all aspects of my personal and professional advocacy for children. As the current chief medical officer for Carolina Complete Health, the only provider-led entity in the active NC Medicaid Transformation to managed care, I continue to witness and thrive upon the energy, talents, insights, and dedication shown by my colleagues at NCPeds. Their contributions to the development of the current Medicaid Transformation Plan and their ability to weather the storms of change have, and will continue to, benefit the citizens of North Carolina in an enduring fashion.

## The View from South Carolina: From Outside Looking In for the Past Quarter Century

by Francis Rushton, MD, FAAP

North Carolinians have much to be proud of in the immense accomplishment of the state's American Academy of Pediatrics (AAP) Chapter (NCPeds). As a South Carolinian, I looked with envy at our northern neighbor's accomplishments. In the early 1990s, District IV included most of what is now District X, running all the way from Dry Tortugas in Florida to Winchester, Virginia; then west across Kentucky and Tennessee to the Ohio and Mississippi Rivers; and then east across the Caribbean to Vieques, Puerto Rico. There was a lot of sharing of idealism across that vast geographic area. But in the early 1990s, I think North Carolina was one of the strongest, if not the strongest, chapters in our district.

Adjoining North Carolina, the state of South Carolina could not help but be influenced by our neighbors. Two North Carolina accomplishments in particular spread elsewhere in the district. The habit that North Carolina developed of sitting down regularly with state officials to consult about child health issues at their open forums was particularly influential, not only in South Carolina but across the American Academy of Pediatrics. In South Carolina we rolled the open forum concept into our winter Community Access to Child Health (CATCH) meeting. This annual gathering has met now for more than a quarter century in downtown Charleston. Portions of the meeting are focused on AAP's CATCH program and South Carolina's ambulatory pediatric quality improvement efforts. But the major portion of the agenda is to provide a forum for state agencies and nonprofits with an interest in child health to interact with the pediatric community, including pediatricians, key pediatric practice staff, and the administrators of the South Carolina chapter.

Although Continuing Medical Education (CME) credit is given, we felt it important to treat all attending as unpaid consultants. We thus have raised funding to pay for the lodging of all who attend each year. South Carolina had nineteen attendees at the winter meeting in 1995 and 180 attendees at our 2020 meeting. Most importantly, South Carolina's version of open forum has catalyzed many efforts that have resulted in child health improvements across our state.

In my opinion, the North Carolina Chapter's second most exportable endeavor has been its legislative advocacy success. Funding a staff person to lobby the state legislature has paid reams of dividends for pediatricians and children alike. As AAP board chair for District IV, I was struck by how successful Tennessee has been with their legislative advocacy using a model like that of North Carolina. North Carolina's contribution to national AAP leadership has been remarkably substantial, not just in Dr. Dave Tayloe Jr.'s and Dr. Steve Edwards' tenures as national presidents but in the efforts of board member Dr. Jane Foy and the service of countless other North Carolinians on AAP committees, sections and councils.

Many North Carolina AAP leaders have additionally impacted our state's child health through their private efforts. There are many but I will mention just a few. Dr. Peter Margolis and Dr. Carol Lannon's healthy development learning collaborative became the prototype for South Carolina's Quality through Technology and Innovation in Pediatrics (QTIP) program. Dr. Olson Huff's success with health systems in Asheville helped inform our own work. Dr. Julie Linton's work with home visitors in Winston-Salem is now reflected in our own eleven federally funded home visitors program housed in South Carolina pediatric offices. Dr. Jane Foy's and Dr. Marian Earl's efforts in Greensboro and with the national Task Force on Mental Health have produced tools and strategies now rolled into our South Carolina QTIP program.

Goldsboro's prodigious community pediatrics work with zero to three initiatives, school health, and others are reflected in our South Carolina Well Baby Plus program in Beaufort and the Greenwood Children's Center. I had the privilege of visiting Dave Tayloe Jr. in Goldsboro in the late 1990s, and wrote about his successes as well as our own in South Carolina.[1]

Under Dave Tayloe Jr.'s guidance, innovative ideas have continued to ensue. Looking from "outside in," North Carolina's achievements have spread. "No one is an island;" neither is a state AAP chapter. Our chapter and others have benefited from North Carolina's successes, and hopefully they have benefited from ours. All the chapters now in the current District IV are among the strongest and most effective in the academy.

## Inspiring the Virginia Chapter to Act for Children

**by Colleen Kraft, MD, FAAP**

The Virginia chapter AAP (VA-AAP) experienced a renaissance at the turn of the 21st Century, largely inspired by the successes of the North Carolina chapter. Tom Sullivan, MD, FAAP, president of the chapter, started a strategic planning process designed to empower pediatricians to organize their efforts to improve conditions for children in the Commonwealth. Virginia saw its neighbor to the south as an innovative center for policies and practices that could launch improvements in care for children and provide infrastructure for pediatricians to start addressing the "new morbidities" of the millennium.

The chapter officers, along with Vice-President Dr. Patricia Reams and Secretary-Treasurer Dr. Les Ellwood, voted first to change the chapter administration. Working with the Richmond Academy of Medicine, the VA-AAP was able to streamline operations. Having seen the successes of North Carolina in state legislative advocacy, the Virginia chapter hired Karen Addison as the first government relations staff. This resulted in Virginia pediatricians successfully working with the legislature

---

[1] Rushton, Francis E. Jr., MD 1998. *Family Support in Community Pediatrics: Confronting New Challenges*. Westport, CT,: Greenwood Publishing Co. (Praeger).

to improve Medicaid payment to physicians serving pregnant women and children; form a statewide immunization registry; improve car seat safety standards; and develop public-private partnerships to support youth tobacco prevention, childhood obesity prevention, and early childhood systems of care. The Pediatric Education Foundation was started to support practice-based education and grant-funded projects for the VA-AAP.

Dr. Pat Reams became VA-AAP chapter president in 2002. Along with chapter Vice President Dr. Les Elwood and Secretary-Treasurer Dr. Colleen Kraft, they fostered improved communication with the Medical Society of Virginia (MSV). The important collaboration of the VA chapter with MSV led to the formation of the first organized resident advocacy day, where pediatric residents statewide gathered to learn the legislative process and speak to state leaders about child health issues. Every January, pediatric residents from five programs (Virginia Commonwealth University, University of Virginia, Children's Hospital of the King's Daughters, Inova Fairfax Hospital, and Virginia Tech Carilion) meet with MSV staff at the capitol and become the voice for Virginia's children in their care. North Carolina had a very close association with its state medical society, utilizing their administrative support until establishing a freestanding office and full-time executive director in 1999.

Virginia pediatricians looked to leaders such as Dr. Chuck Willson, who, with the Community Care of North Carolina program, launched quality improvement programs in the management of asthma in children. Dr. Jane Foy and Dr. Marian Earls were leaders in addressing behavioral health concerns in children, utilizing concrete tools and pathways for primary care pediatricians to start screening, evaluating, and treating children. Dr. Dave Tayloe Jr. and his practice at Goldsboro Pediatrics showed how pediatricians in an underserved community could work within that community and partner with hospitals, school-based health care centers, and local nonprofit organizations to enhance care for all children.

Drs. Steve Edwards and Dave Tayloe Jr., former AAP presidents from North Carolina, promoted the idea that pediatricians need appropriate payment for child health services, especially for children with Medicaid. They emphasized that payment was important to "ensure that there is always a pediatrician in the community, on the ground, who can care for a child." One significant win for pediatricians in Virginia came in 2007, when the General Assembly, along with Medicaid Director Pat Finnerty, voted for a significant increase in Medicaid payment for pediatric and obstetric services. This opened access for many more children in Virginia, as pediatricians could make the margin to support their mission. The inspiration for this work came from our North Carolina colleagues.

North Carolina pediatricians encouraged us to get involved in the state legislature through the open forum concept. Where Virginia did not adopt that specific program,

## The Virginia chapter AAP (VA-AAP) experienced a renaissance at the turn of the 21st Century, largely inspired by the successes of the North Carolina chapter.

our chapter has developed considerable influence on how the Commonwealth operates for child health. One story from the Virginia legislature that continues to emphasize the importance of pediatricians speaking to elected leaders concerned the requirement of the Tdap vaccine for entry into sixth grade. Senator Janet Howell introduced the legislation. She was met with the question from the Senate Health and Education Committee, "What about the mercury in those vaccines?" Her answer? "Oh, we are not talking about vaccines; we are talking about immunizations!" The Senate Health and Education Committee then voted out the bill 15-0 without any members realizing that immunizations are vaccines! Fortunately, the next year, Dr. Ralph Northam, a child neurologist from Norfolk, was elected to the Virginia State Senate. The Senate Health and Education Committee finally had its own pediatric expert. Dr. Northam became lieutenant governor of Virginia in 2014 and was sworn in as Virginia's 73rd governor of the Commonwealth on January 13, 2018.

The Virginia AAP chapter leaders continue to take innovative ideas from the North Carolina chapter to significantly influence policies, laws, and programs that affect children. Chapter Presidents Drs. Bob Gunther, Bill Moskowitz, Biff Reese, Barbara Kahler, Sam Bartle, Sandy Chung, and now Mike Martin have been at the helm of programs inspired by North Carolina, such as Virginia's H1N1 and COVID-19 response; Quality Improvement programs to improve HPV immunization rates; the development of the Virginia Mental Health Access Project (VMAP); and a robust pediatric education program. VA-AAP Executive Director Jane Chappell, who coordinated many of these activities, now serves as the grant manager for VA-AAP. Of note, three past presidents of VA-AAP were elected as national AAP president: Dr. Joe Zanga (1997-98), Dr. Colleen Kraft (2018-19), and Dr. Sandy Chung (2023-24).

Dr. Tom Sullivan, who was a visionary in his reorganization of the Virginia chapter, died tragically in 2014 when he was accidentally struck by a vehicle while crossing the street. His legacy lives on in the Virginia chapter leadership, in the programs that help pediatricians support families, and in the interaction with elected leaders in

Virginia to make positive changes for children. The Virginia chapter still looks to North Carolina for its pediatricians' creativity, enthusiasm, and programs that help pediatricians better care for their patients.

## NCPeds Memories from Wisconsin

by Kathy Nichol, MD, MS, FAAP

When I was president of the Wisconsin chapter of the American Academy of Pediatrics in the early 90s, the academy held an annual meeting, later named the National Conference and Exhibition (NCE). It also convened a chapter forum (later named the Annual Leadership Forum, abbreviated ALF), where all of the AAP chapter presidents and vice presidents were invited. During that meeting, announcements were made as to which small, medium, large, and then extra-large chapters deserved awards for their advocacy work. I do not remember all the specific projects the NC chapter implemented to win those awards frequently and to improve the health of children in their state, but I remember the liaison committee/open forum infrastructure they utilized to make it happen, which was a very unusual format at the time.

> NCPeds has created a culture, and probably a legacy, that always needs to be tended because it has become the model for the state and a wider audience.

In 1993, I accepted a position as vice president of medical affairs at a community hospital in Milwaukee. I hoped to utilize some of what I learned about leadership when obtaining my master of science (MS) degree. NCPeds exemplified so many of those principles, particularly incorporating the input of stakeholders when attempting to make changes. NC utilized not only the thoughts and ideas of its members but also those of academics, public health professionals, families, and many other stakeholders, depending on the project. They also had the benefit of pediatric leaders who, by nature, were very collaborative.

I worked most closely with Dr. Steve Edwards and Dr. Dave Tayloe Jr. during those years, and it is a great advantage to have leaders who grasp the importance of these principles. Their leadership qualities were well understood by the membership as both were presidents of the AAP later in their careers. Both were particularly good listeners and respected everyone's viewpoint. I think these are also important qualities that enhance the process. The AAP had leadership conferences in the past for potential future leaders. I do not know if that still exists, but I think they are invaluable for helping give skills to up-and-coming leaders. NCPeds has created a culture, and probably a legacy, that always needs to be tended because it has become the model for the state and a wider audience. It reminds me of those magical teams that appear every once in a while, where the chemistry, the skill sets, and the leadership all come together to create something greater than the individual parts. I hope NCPeds can continue to thrive and "export" its experiences to others in the AAP.

# Appendix

SPECIAL ARTICLE

# Working to Improve Mental Health Services: The North Carolina Advocacy Effort

Jane Meschan Foy, MD*; Marian F. Earls, MD‡; and David A. Horowitz, MD§

ABSTRACT. Poor reimbursement of pediatricians for behavioral and developmental services and the disarray of children's mental health services in the state led leaders of the North Carolina chapter of the American Academy of Pediatrics to organize an advocacy effort with the following objectives: 1) to articulate pediatricians' perspective on the current crisis in delivering and coordinating children's behavioral health services; 2) to represent the collective voice of both academic and community pediatricians in dialogue with mental health providers, Medicaid leaders, and the health and mental health segments of state government; 3) to build consensus about an achievable plan of action to address pediatricians' reimbursement and systems issues; 4) to develop a full and appropriate role for pediatricians as providers and, potentially, coordinators of behavioral health care; and 5) to facilitate implementation of Medicaid changes, as a first step in carrying out this plan. This article describes the 24-month process that achieved these objectives. *Pediatrics* 2002;110:1232–1237; *mental health, advocacy, Medicaid.*

## NORTH CAROLINA'S SETTING AS DESCRIBED IN DECEMBER 1998

In North Carolina (NC), as in many other states, mental health (MH) services are in disarray. Inadequate reimbursement has undermined the capacity of virtually every source of MH care, with the end result being that children of all income levels have limited access to behavioral health services. Many communities have no child psychiatrists and an inadequate number of MH providers trained and credentialed to care for children. Medicaid's low reimbursement for office visits, requirement of a definitive diagnosis, and lack of reimbursement for the many nonface-to-face aspects of delivering behavioral health services have contributed significantly to many providers' reluctance or inability to serve publicly insured children.

---

ABBREVIATIONS. NC, North Carolina; MH, mental health; AAP, American Academy of Pediatrics; SCHIP, State Children's Health Insurance Program; SHP, state health plan; DMA, Division of Medical Assistance.

---

From the *Department of Pediatrics, Wake Forest University School of Medicine, Winston-Salem, North Carolina; ‡UNC-Chapel Hill, the Moses H. Cone Memorial Hospital Pediatric Teaching Program and Guilford Child Health, Greensboro, North Carolina; and §UNC-Chapel Hill, Triangle Pediatric Center, Cary, North Carolina.

Received for publication Jan 29, 2002; accepted Jun 12, 2002.

Address correspondence to Jane Meschan Foy, MD, Department of Pediatrics, Wake Forest University School of Medicine, Medical Center Blvd, Winston-Salem, NC 27157.

Table 1, an excerpt from the position paper developed as a tool in NC's advocacy effort, provides an example. Disparate deductibles, co-payments, and caps for MH services in private health plans have created access barriers for privately insured children as well.

Primary care pediatricians, faced with these barriers and with the estimated 30% of children who require MH intervention,[1] frequently experience pressure to prescribe psychiatric medications and deliver services for which they feel inadequately trained. Some have attempted to expand their expertise and involve themselves in these new areas. Others, already frustrated by inadequate compensation for the many behavioral services they provide in the context of comprehensive pediatric care, refer children with behavioral problems through available channels, knowing that only 21% of children with MH problems receive MH services,[2] 70% to 80% of these through the meager resources of public schools,[2] where MH professionals are focused primarily on testing and attendance issues.

In NC, as elsewhere in the country, there is an artificial schism between behavioral health systems and medical systems of care. Poor coordination and poor integration of MH services with children's pediatric care further diminish accessibility and quality of the care that is provided in both the public and private sectors. Inadequately funded public MH facilities experience high turnover of staff and difficulty with recruitment; those MH professionals who are on staff usually are anonymous to community pediatricians. Because NC Medicaid does not allow social workers and psychologists to bill Medicaid unless they are employed or credentialed by a statefunded, state-administered MH program, collegial relationships between pediatricians and Medicaid MH providers are virtually nonexistent in most communities. In many private health plans, families selfrefer children for behavioral services; here also there are often inadequate or absent procedures for communication between MH providers and primary care physicians, who often do not have access to the list of behavioral health providers. Reimbursement for MH services is frequently allowed only to MH providers, eliminating any financial incentive for primary care physicians to share in the care of children with MH conditions.

For all these reasons, pediatricians are frequently unaware of medications prescribed by MH providers and of therapeutic efforts important to the ongoing management of a child's emotional and family problems. An additional factor contributing to poor coordination is the paucity of care coordination programs in NC for children with behavioral problems and mental illness: the state-funded Child Services Coordination Program serves children with developmental and medical problems from birth to age 5; neither the Child Services Coordination Progam nor the state-supported Developmental Evaluation Centers serve school-aged children. Low ratios of school nurses in the state—1:2451 statewide, 1:5000 or more in some

| **TABLE 1. Excerpt from the NC Pediatric Society Position Paper** | | | |
| --- | --- | --- | --- |
| | Medicaid to Pediatrician in Private Practice | Private Plan 1 | Private Plan 2 |
| Current Procedural Terminology Code 99205, comprehensive, new patient | $114.21 | $128.00 | $148.50 |

The pediatrician spent 120 minutes evaluating a hyperkinetic 7-year old, implementing and coordinating therapy for attention-deficit/hyperactivity disorder, writing reports, and following up by telephone. If this had been an established patient instead of a new patient, the Medicaid reimbursement would have been lower still.

areas[3]—prevent most nurses from playing a role in coordination. Public school psychologists and guidance counselors, who deliver the majority of MH services to youth,[2] function virtually outside the health care system.

Compounding these reimbursement and coordination issues in NC, as elsewhere, are the problems arising from the compartmentalized training of MH and medical professionals and the separate administrative structures that perpetuate this compartmentalization. As a result, MH professionals and community pediatricians typically do not work in the same buildings, utilize the same terminology or diagnostic approach, attend the same educational programs, use the same forms or reimbursement codes, or sit at the same tables to address their concerns. At the level of state government, 2 separate systems, functioning largely in parallel and funded by separate streams, oversee medical programs in 1 building, MHprograms in another. This separation posed significant challenges for the process of addressing NC's problems.

## NC'S ASSETS

NC has an active chapter of the American Academy of Pediatrics (AAP) and 5 academic pediatric programs whose chairs are closely involved in the chapter's educational and advocacy efforts. The chapter has a long history of effective collaboration with state government, enhanced by the tenure of David Bruton, MD, a community pediatrician from Pinehurst, North Carolina, who served as secretary of the Department of Health and Human Services from 1997–2001. The primary setting for the chapter's collaboration has been an open forum, convened 3 times yearly by the chapter, which brings together pediatricians, child advocates, and representatives of state government to update each other on important developments affecting the health of children and to address mutual concerns. The former Director of Medicaid, Richard Perruzzi, was among the attendees. Secretary Bruton and

Mr. Perruzzi worked closely with chapter leaders in developing a non-Medicaid State Children's Health Insurance Program (SCHIP) built around the State Health Plan (SHP) for state employees. The SHP experience in MH coverage had been especially positive: in 1992, NC introduced into the SHP full coverage parity of MH and non-MH conditions, a single insurance deductible, full freedom of choice of MH providers, and only moderate management of generous benefits through a contract with Value Behavioral Health. With MH parity in place, by 1998 NC had seen the following changes[4]:

→ MH payments as a percentage of total health payments decreased from 6.4% to 3.1%.

→ MH hospital days decreased by 70%.

→ Actual per member/per month cost for MH benefits (including administrative overhead) went from $5.43 in fiscal year 1990 to $4.11 in fiscal year 1998.

→ Actual utilization patterns remained constant and modest: 6% to 7% of enrollees sought outpatient services per year; half went for only 3 to 4 sessions, three-fourths completed treatment within 11 to 13 sessions; utilization > 26 visits remained constant and low (0.40%–0.75%).

Although MH parity did not increase overall costs, and although it brought about a marked reduction in inpatient MH days (an outcome also documented by Sturm, who studied insurance plans that offered parity in behavioral health spending limits[5]), these data were insufficient to persuade state legislators to pass MH parity legislation on multiple annual attempts. However, the SHP experience was sufficient to open dialogue that could not have otherwise occurred in NC's fiscally conservative political climate.

## THE PROCESS

### 1) Articulating Pediatricians' Perspective: The Position Paper

A critical first step was bringing together pediatricians to form a task force of NC's AAP chapter. Key members felt passionate about the MH issue, had expertise and experience, and were already involved in chapter leadership: a community pediatrician who chairs the chapter's Mental Health Committee and is the parent of a child with special developmental needs; an academic developmentalist from the chapter's Committee on Disabilities; a developmental pediatrician who serves as medical director of a community health program for low-income children in an urban county, former chair of the local Board of Mental Health, Developmental Disabilities, and Substance Abuse, and Chair of the chapter's School Health Committee; and an adolescent specialist in combined community and academic practice, former chair of the chapter's Committee on Adolescence. The chair of the group, which was named the Task Force on Mental Health Care Access and Reimbursement, is an academic generalist, formerly in private and public health settings, involved in developing school-based health services and serving as NC's AAP chapter president.

As the group began meeting to discuss the problem, anecdotal experiences and discussion about our sources of frustration dominated the discussion. It became evident that, to move forward, we needed to find expression for the angst, educate each other about unfamiliar aspects of the issues, and prepare to speak in one, understandable voice to fellow child advocates and policymakers. We settled on the idea of writing a position paper, which went through many iterations and served to focus our efforts during our first few months. This document appears on the Web site of the NC chapter of the AAP, which is available at: www.ncpeds.org.

## 2) Including Other Stakeholders: Consensus Plan

Having reached consensus on the position paper, we began expanding our Task Force to include other MH advocates, including the executive directors of the state's organizations for social workers, psychologists, and psychiatrists and the president of the state's Council of Child and Adolescent Psychiatrists. These individuals brought with them their experience in lobbying the state legislature and state government on MH issues, linkage to other advocacy groups such as the Alliance for the Mentally Ill, and their own expressions of anger and frustration, which the Task Force processed and discussed over several meetings. With their input, the Task Force developed a plan of action, which served mutual goals; this plan became a second chapter of the position paper, which is available at: www.ncpeds.org.

## 3) Working With Medicaid

With this document complete, we made the decision to approach Medicaid leadership. The group's optimism was greatly increased by a surprise legislative response to years of chapter advocacy, facilitated by Secretary Bruton, to increase Medicaid rates to parity with Medicare, effective January 1, 1999, and to allow clients 1 year of Medicaid eligibility, rather than month-to-month. Although these measures were not specific to MH and did not solve other problems, such as the absence of reimbursement for nonface-to-face activities and barriers to collaboration with Medicaid MH providers, they were enormously helpful to the cause and signaled a mood of receptiveness to physician concerns.

The Task Force approached the Director of Medicaid, and he agreed to meet with the group about its access and reimbursement concerns. We decided to locate the meeting in his conference room at the Division of Medical Assistance (DMA) building and have met there regularly since, frequently involving other members of the DMA staff and consulting with them about wording of new regulations resulting from our negotiations, as well as unrelated topics such as preventive dental programs, for which they needed our advice and support. We soon pulled in other members of state government, leaders from the Department of Mental Health, Developmental Disabilities and Substance Abuse Services, who had not previously interacted with our pediatric leadership, and began to address MH systems issues, as well as reimbursement. These new relationships continue to be of great value to the chapter.

## 4) Outcomes

Advocacy is not science; consequently, outcomes cannot be attributed tidily to any 1 factor in the complex environment of that period. Generations of chapter leaders gave this advocacy effort their legacy of credibility and effective relationships with state government. Secretary Bruton's powerful position and supportive posture toward the Task Force undoubtedly helped to get Medicaid leaders to the table and to facilitate progress. Other MH advocacy groups worked in parallel with the Task Force, invigorated by the support of pediatricians. To these ingredients the Task Force added focus, persistence, a consensus voice, a framework for negotiation, and access to the clinical expertise of pediatricians motivated to participate in a change effort.

Results came about laboriously. Several contentious issues required discussions by telephone or in small groups outside Task Force meetings. Occasionally, impacted groups (eg, physicians in local area MH programs) requested a hearing of their concerns, which were all heard first by Task Force representatives, then considered and addressed by the Task Force as a whole. Meticulous notes of meetings (an essential component of an advocacy effort) recorded agreements and reminded the group of unfinished business. Snags sometimes required data-gathering, outside expertise, and special visitors to Task Force meetings, occasionally including Secretary Bruton himself or other members of the Department of Health and Human Services staff. Periodically, the Task Force revised the position paper to clarify a point and then recirculated it to Secretary Bruton and other government leaders.

The following Medicaid changes resulted from this collaborative effort:

✔ Reimbursement for up to 6 visits to a MH/ substance abuse provider without assigning a diagnosis and up to 26 unmanaged visits in a calendar year for Medicaid recipients up to age 21.[6] DMA confirmed on October 12, 2001 that this policy also applies to physicians performing behavioral assessment and treatment.

✔ [a]**Primary care provider referral for up to 26 MH visits annually for children under the age of 21.**[7] MH providers are educated to communicate at regular intervals with the primary care provider.

✔ **Expansion of "incident to" rules,**[b] **allowing physicians employing licensed clinical social workers, and clinical nurse specialists with psychiatric certification to bill for the services of these MH professionals if the physician provides on-site supervision.**[8]

✓ Expansion of "incident to" rules,[b] allowing health departments who employ licensed clinical social workers, licensed psychologists, and advanced practice nurses to bill for their services in schoolbased health centers, if a physician provides supervision by phone or beeper.[9]

✓ **[a]Direct Medicaid enrollment of independently practicing licensed clinical social workers, licensed psychologists, and advanced practice nurses allowing them to bill for services delivered in their offices.**[10,11,12]

✓ An additional provision allowing independently enrolled MH professionals to bill for services delivered in school sites.[13]

We were not successful in achieving Medicaid reimbursement for nonface-to-face services. Nor were we successful in achieving an enhanced fee for services performed by pediatricians with subspecialty training. Both these approaches created troubling complications for DMA outside the realm of pediatrics. Although we were successful in enabling new categories of MH professionals to deliver services in school sites without on-site physician supervision, we were unsuccessful in expanding this opportunity to those employed by private physicians or universities.

We should add that some of these changes created new challenges for NC's area MH programs. For the first time, they must compete for physician referrals of low-income patients. A positive outcome has been their heightened interest in streamlining their own referral processes and enhancing communication with referring physicians. A negative outcome has been the growing phenomenon of split therapy, a name they have given to the circumstance that develops when a nonphysician community MH professional delivers a portion of a patient's therapy and a physician without an established relationship with that professional is expected to deliver the other (eg, emergency hospitalization or psychopharmacologic therapy). The latter problem appears amenable to relationship-building among the concerned parties and may prove an additional incentive to collaboration.

## 5) Educating Our Membership

To bring the membership of our chapter along in the process and to expand pediatricians' capacity to deliver and coordinate behavioral and MH services, we planned educational sessions around the topics our Task Force identified as most critical, including developmental and behavioral health screening, psychopharmacology, and

---

[a]We anticipate that the steps in bold print will facilitate pediatricians' collegial relationships with, employment of, and/or co-location with MH professionals. We believe that these changes will, in turn, improve access to MH services for Medicaid-enrolled children and increase the likelihood that these services will be provided within or coordinated with a child's medical home.

[b]"Incident to" rules govern billing for services delivered by a physician's employee in the name of the physician. Before August 2000, NC's rules restricted "incident to" billing to PhD psychologists. Before September 2000, NC's rules required the physician to be on-site at the time the employee delivered the service.

coding for MH services and special needs health care. The session on coding received the highest evaluation of any offering. Future offerings will focus on expansion of other MH skills important to primary care pediatricians: use of the Diagnostic and *Statistical Manual for Primary Care*, family assessment, management of attention-deficit/hyperactivity disorder and depression, collaboration with schools and other community agencies, referral to MH professionals, and behavioral therapy.

We met with the leadership of our NC area health education centers to plan regional grand rounds on MH topics. NC's Council of Child and Adolescent Psychiatrists is participating in this effort. The Northwest Area Health Education Center, which serves 17 counties, has undertaken a project to assist selected communities in organizing systems of care for children with attention problems. This effort will be patterned after a successful model in Guilford County, which developed a community protocol for the assessment of children with classroom inattention and behavior problems; established roles for school personnel, public health nurses, primary physicians, and MH agencies in the assessment and management of these children; created communication forms and procedures for each step of these processes; and implemented an educational plan for introducing these new procedures to physicians and school personnel.

The next phase of our educational effort will be workshops for pediatricians on collaboration with MH providers, explaining new reimbursement opportunities. We will be distributing the names of newly enrolled MH providers (400 statewide as of this writing), information about their training and scope of practice, and recommended referral procedures. A new brochure under development by NC's representatives on the AAP's Committee on Psychosocial Aspects of Child and Family Health will facilitate this process.

### 6) Other Advocacy Efforts

The chapter joined with our colleagues in social work, psychology, and psychiatry for yet another failed effort to pass legislation requiring parity of MH benefits in insurance plans. Our chapter's resolution to address MH parity specifically in the AAP's Universal Health Insurance proposal was passed by the 2000 AAP Annual Chapter Forum. Our chapter's resolution to provide assistance to chapters on MH issues was adopted by the 2001 Annual Chapter Forum.

Private insurers lag well behind in improving MH benefits. The chapter formed a group, the Managed Care Solutions Committee, to move the chapter's advocacy efforts into the private sector. Medical directors of NC's major managed care organizations meet to discuss an agenda that is jointly developed by our chapter leadership and a health maintenance organization medical director, who is also a pediatrician. Modest first steps in relation to MH include an agreement to share behavioral health provider lists with pediatricians and attention-deficit/hyperactivity disorder coding guidelines specific to each of the plans.

Perhaps the Task Force's most long-lasting accomplishment will be the inclusion of pediatricians on state government committees and MH planning groups that previously did not include any primary care physicians.

### NEXT STEPS

There is much left to do. Evaluation of NC's progress toward improving access to MH services for Medicaid-enrolled children will be a challenge. Medicaid has only claims data. In these data, MH services delivered by employed MH professionals under new "incident to" policies are so far indistinguishable from those delivered by their supervising physicians. On the other hand, we will be able to track the number and type of services delivered by newly enrolled independent providers and the total number of MH services delivered. Individual providers will be able to analyze their changes in reimbursement. Other measures will require a separate evaluation effort.

We remain hopeful that improvements in Medicaid will place pressure on private insurers if and when we achieve a buy-in option for children who are financially ineligible for Medicaid and SCHIP. If, as we suspect from experience in the SHP, improved MH benefits in Medicaid and SCHIP do not have adverse cost implications, there may be incentives for expanding private MH benefits, even without the buy-in option.

### LESSONS LEARNED ABOUT WORKING WITH STATE GOVERNMENT

The following principles drawn from NC's experience may be helpful to pediatricians in their advocacy efforts:

1. Advocates must take advantage of political opportunities that present themselves. One such opportunity is a sympathetic person in a key government role; this might be a physician, a parent, or grandparent of a child with mental illness, or a child advocate. Full advantage is gained only if pediatricians with the requisite clinical expertise position themselves to be accessible and well-organized during this person's period of empowerment, with clearly articulated consensus positions on important policy areas.

2. State government administrators often view subspecialty care, especially that which is delivered at academic centers, as exotic and expensive. There may also be an adversarial relationship between the governmental agency and the medical center. Efforts by academic pediatricians to lobby state government on their own behalf appear self-serving and suffer from this baggage. Academic pediatricians will benefit from joining with community pediatricians in their AAP state chapter to approach Medicaid and other state agencies. The community pediatrician can

speak to the value of subspecialty services in the care of their patients. This reframes the academicians' problems in terms of access to care for children in need, rather than survival of tertiary hospital infrastructure (a cause that few government officials will find appealing).

3. Personal relationships with state government leaders are at the heart of successful negotiations. These grow over time. Many AAP state chapters have developed these relationships over a long period, adding to their value as partners in any advocacy effort. Parents and grandparents of patients may also have relationships with administrators or with legislators, as well as passion and experience to bring to an advocacy effort.

4. State government leaders weary of listening to splinter perspectives of various advocacy groups. All advocates are best served by participating in a coalition, which agrees on a common agenda. If there are issues outside this common agenda— especially if they are in conflict with the common agenda— there should be advance understanding by all partners in the coalition. One partner's end run around a process and agenda developed by a coalition is very destructive to trust and credibility.

5. A government official will have little sympathy for enhancing physicians' income, especially because it probably far exceeds his own. The fundamental issue when seeking increased reimbursement should always be access. The AAP Members Only Channel provides links to a number of documents that make the case for the association between access and reimbursement (available at: www.aap.org/moc/medlegal2.CFM).

6. Child advocates must seek out opportunities to understand the perspective of state government administrators and, when possible, to assist them with their problems. Frequently, these opportunities enable advocates to address their own concerns in an unexpected way. In the present economic environment, opportunities for cost-saving are particularly powerful. The state DMA will likely have a medical director—possibly a pediatrician— who is a good initial contact. By linking DMA to pediatricians with expertise in the management of complex and expensive conditions, advocates can assist Medicaid in reducing cost and improving quality, while laying the groundwork for a productive problem-solving relationship.

7. Child advocates must pursue strategies that are compatible with the political and economic environment. Administrators of state government agencies serve political leaders. They are looking for opportunities to align themselves with their constituents' interests.

8. Specific strategies most beneficial in negotiating with Medicaid will necessarily vary from state to state. The following section suggests some approaches that may yield results.

## APPROACHES TO MEDICAID

The exact approach a state uses to negotiate with Medicaid will depend on the particular shortcomings of that Medicaid program. Examples might include the following:

- Codes reimbursed by Medicare but not Medicaid
- Absence of reimbursement for visits not resulting in a diagnostic code (ie, screening, testing, multivisit assessment)
- Absence of reimbursement for nonface-to-face services (telephone consultation, record review, parent or school conferences, etc)
- Restrictions built into the "incident to" policy (supervision requirements, failure to reimburse categories of MH professionals)
- Impediments to reimbursement for MH services delivered on school premises
- Failure to recognize advanced credentials of physicians (ie, no enhanced fee for a more complex service delivered by a more highly trained professional)
- Failure to reimburse categories of MH professionals and MH professionals in certain employment arrangements
- Monopolies of state MH programs
- Managed care policies excluding the primary care physician from referral/management decisions
- Monthly renewal of Medicaid eligibility (as opposed to yearly)
- Across-the-board inadequacies in reimbursement

The negotiation process involves exploring the feasibility of each of these strategies with Medicaid leaders. Some will have more appeal than others, depending on that Medicaid agency's history and political climate. Child advocates dealing with tight state budgets must fight the perception that increasing access will balloon costs. NC's experience with its SHP (see above) and the experience of other plans that provide MH parity6 contradict this perception: total expenditures for MH care have, at most, modestly increased with parity; furthermore, plans with parity have experienced the very positive outcome of decreased inpatient days. There are undoubtedly other needed MH care reforms, such as those that build the capacity of neglected systems, that will be financially costly; advocates for these changes must build their case around the human and economic costs of untreated behavioral problems.

### REFERENCES

1. *Comprehensive Child Health Plan: 2000–2005. Report to the North Carolina Department of Health and Human Services.* Chapel Hill, NC: North Carolina Institute of Medicine; May 23, 2000:86
2. Burns BJ, Costello EJ, Angold A, et al. Children's mental health service use across service sectors. *Health Aff.* 1995;14:147–159
3. *Comprehensive Child Health Plan: 2000–2005. Report to the North Carolina Department of Health and Human Services.* Chapel Hill, NC: North Carolina Institute of Medicine; May 23, 2000:77

4. Data on the Mental Health Benefit. Prepared by the North Carolina Psychological Association from data supplied by the North Carolina State Health Plan Office. April 1999

5. Sturm R. How expensive is unlimited mental health coverage under managed care? *JAMA.* 1997;278:1533–1537

6. A new health benefit. *NC Medicaid Bulletin.* June 2000:13

7. Referral policy for specialty care. *NC Medicaid Bulletin.* August 2001:4

8. Incident to policy for licensed clinical social workers and clinical nurse specialists. *NC Medicaid Bulletin.* August 2000:14

9. Supervision of services performed in health departments. *NC Medicaid Bulletin* September 2000:21

10. Independent mental health provider seminars. *NC Medicaid Bulletin.* January 2001:46

11. Outpatient mental health services for children birth through 20 years of age. *NC Medicaid Bulletin.* February 2001:2

12. Credentialing requirements—correction to terminology in January 2001 Medicaid special bulletin I, provider enrollment guidelines. *NC Medicaid Bulletin.* March 2001:18

13. Place of service for outpatient therapy. *NC Medicaid Bulletin.* September 2001:11

## WORKING TEENAGERS

"American teenagers are an atypically industrious lot. In most developed countries, teenagers work only if the family needs income. Yet the American teens most likely to work have historically been white, and (perhaps most surprisingly of all) had a family income above $40,000 a year. By contrast, poor inner-city kids have been much less likely to hold jobs. A new report by the Center for Labor Market Studies at Northeastern University in Boston points out that this has been the toughest summer-job market for teenagers in 37 years."

*The Economist.* August 24, 2002
Noted by JFL, MD

# AAP Resident "Community Access to Child Health" (CATCH) Grants to North Carolina 2017-2022

**By Debra Best, MD, FAAP**

NCPeds has supported Community Access to Child Health (CATCH) grants from the American Academy of Pediatrics for individual pediatric residents and joint projects. Some of these have made advocacy the theme for securing policy change. There are five examples of North Carolina pediatric residents' CATCH grant projects featuring advocacy in the appendix.

The AAP CATCH Program offers residents and practicing pediatricians the opportunity to pursue collaborative projects within their communities that aim to provide access to services that support the health and well-being of children. For residents who are particularly interested in advocacy, CATCH grants provide a wonderful entry point to bring resources to bear on the development and support of innovative community partnerships to address unmet needs. Grants are intended to focus on building strong partnerships in the community and on serving those who are underserved and/or experience health disparities.

Since 2017, North Carolina applicants have been awarded twelve resident CATCH grants for services and ten planning/implementation CATCH grants.

I served as NC Chapter CATCH Facilitator from 2010-2023. My role was to provide guidance and technical support to pediatric residents and practicing pediatricians as they pursued grant funding for community-related endeavors. Current NCPeds CATCH facilitators are Aaron Pankiewicz, DO (Cary), and Larissa Truschel, MD, MPH (Durham).

## INJURY & VIOLENCE: TOOLKIT FOR PREVENTING DOG BITE INJURIES

AAP CATCH Grant/Residents – 2017

Contacts: Sarah Duffus, MD; Jordan Norris, MD

University of North Carolina School of Medicine, Chapel Hill

### PROGRAM DESCRIPTION

The primary aim of this project is to reduce the number of life-threatening dog bite injuries sustained by children in our community. The number of pediatric trauma patients treated at our tertiary care center, the North Carolina Children's Hospital at the University of North Carolina (UNC), for injuries caused by dog bites more than doubled from 2013 through 2016. Very few resources currently exist to assist in the reduction of injuries in children less than five years old. We created a task force at UNC that has partnered with the NC State College of Veterinary Medicine to create evidence-based educational materials for use in both primary care pediatrics and veterinary office settings. The pediatric resident members of the task force are committed to the following:

1. Working with our veterinary colleagues to create a "provider toolkit" of evidenced-based educational materials in both print and video form. Materials will include data to inform pediatricians about the scope of the problem and how to counsel patients, in addition to educational handouts for families. Similar resources will be created specifically for use in veterinary offices, and will include tools for connecting families to a medical home if their child does not currently have a primary care pediatrician.

2. Evaluating the toolkit resources for the quality of their use in the primary care pediatrics setting.

3. Making these resources widely available to pediatricians in our surrounding community and throughout the state of North Carolina.

4. Creating an online database for PCPs to report dog bite injuries and assess tetanus immunization status of the injured patient.

**GOALS**

1. To create a comprehensive "provider toolkit" of information related to dog bite injury prevention, containing both print and audio-visual materials for use by primary care pediatricians during birth to five-year well visits and by veterinarians caring for dogs owned by families with children.

2. To make the toolkit available to all primary care pediatric practices and veterinary offices in Orange County, North Carolina. Also, to disseminate the toolkit to at least fifty other pediatric practices throughout North Carolina using the NC Pediatric Society annual meeting and e-mail listserv.

3. To establish and maintain a database for collection of dog bite injury data being treated in the outpatient setting so that the scope of this problem may be better understood.

## NUTRITION: BULL CITY BOOKS AND BITES

**AAP CATCH Grant/Residents – 2018**

**Contact: Jennifer Lawson, MD**

**Duke Children's Primary Care – Duke University Medical Center, Durham**

### PROGRAM DESCRIPTION

Food insecurity is defined by the US Department of Agriculture as any household in which access to adequate food is limited by a lack of money or other resources. Data reveals that 19.1 percent of the population of Durham County experience food insecurity, and, of children under the age of eighteen, some 20.1 percent are food insecure. Within our primary care clinic, preliminary chart review data indicate that 30 percent of patients and families are food insecure. Food insecurity has significant potential health consequences, including developmental delay, behavioral issues, and chronic medical conditions such as diabetes and cardiovascular disease.

To combat this concern, we have partnered with Durham Public Schools and the Durham Public Library to enhance an already established, yet underutilized, summer food program for those in need. We will offer a food pantry to complement this program, as well as education and enrichment resources, such as books, reading, art, and music. We aim to increase the utilization of the current meal program and enhance nutritional support for these children throughout the year. In addition, we will use this opportunity to better serve our community by screening children for medical homes, medical insurance, and immunization status. We will offer resource support to those identified with needs in these areas.

### GOALS

The goals are:

1. Distribute per family one to two boxes of supplemental food each week during school breaks, beginning during the summer of 2018, at the T. A. Grady Community Center in Durham in conjunction with the Durham Public Library.

2. Screen and provide access to appropriate insurance, medical home, and vaccines to 100 percent of pediatric participants during school breaks beginning in the summer of 2018.

3. Increase participation in summer and fall break meal programs offered by the Durham Public Library to the Durham community by 100 percent by providing additional supplemental food in a literacy-rich environment.

## BREASTFEEDING: INCREASING ACCESS TO BREAST PUMPS

**AAP CATCH Grant/Residents – 2019**

**Contact: India Hanvey, MD**

**University of North Carolina School of Medicine, Chapel Hill**

### PROGRAM DESCRIPTION

The primary aim is to develop sustainable, collaborative relationships with community partners to answer the question: "How do we increase access to electric breast pumps for underserved mothers in our community, especially during the first month of breastfeeding?" Our second goal is to assess common barriers to breastfeeding that mothers experience in our local community, including Orange and Durham counties.

A 2012 *PEDIATRICS* article showed that 85 percent of women who deliver in breastfeeding-friendly hospitals plan to breastfeed their infants for the first three months of life. However, only 32 percent ever reach their goal. In North Carolina, the percentage of breastfeeding infants drops to approximately 26 percent at six months of life, according to the 2018 NC Child Health Report Card by the Institute of Medicine and NC Child. Early return to work, latch problems, and the need for nipple stimulation are common barriers that can be improved with electric pumps. Private-insured patients are often eligible for pumps prenatally. However, Medicaid-insured patients receive electric pumps from the Women, Infants and Children (WIC) Program only after exclusively breastfeeding for one month. Very few resources exist to provide electric pumps immediately postpartum.

Our resident team commits to achieve the following:

1. Evaluate barriers to breastfeeding in our community through two focus groups with nursing mothers and through surveys distributed at outpatient lactation appointments.
2. Facilitate two collaborative meetings between lactation consultants, breastfeeding mothers, the Women's Birth and Wellness Center (WBWC), Women's Health Information Center (WHICH), Piedmont Health Services (FQHC), Orange County WIC program, and pediatric residents to discuss community breastfeeding barriers.
3. Design a sustainable, community-based system that increases access to electric breast pumps among WIC-eligible breastfeeding mothers.
4. Pilot a prepaid voucher system that allows at least twenty WIC-eligible mothers to exchange prepaid vouchers for a one-week to one-month breast pump rental at the Women's Birth and Wellness Center. A temporary breast pump rental will bridge the gap between infant delivery and a mother's eligibility for an electric pump at one month.

The primary setting for the project will be the Women's Birth and Wellness Center (WBWC), a community organization committed to providing maternity and postpartum health care. WBWC will provide a safe space for collaborative meetings with the community partners, as well as a comfortable place for focus groups with local breastfeeding mothers. WBWC will also be the primary site for piloting a prepaid voucher system for one-week to one-month breast pump rentals.

## GOALS

1. Collect 100 surveys from nursing mothers who attend lactation appointments or infant well-child checks (<12 months of age) at the WBWC, WIC, or UNC lactation outpatient 26/36 clinics (UNC Children's Primary Care or UNC pediatrics at Panther Creek).
2. Schedule and facilitate two 2-hour collaborative meetings with community partners to review the most prominent community breastfeeding barriers that were identified through the surveys and focus groups previously described.
3. Provide at least twenty Medicaid- or WIC-eligible breastfeeding mothers with a prepaid voucher they can exchange for a one-week electric breast pump rental at the WBWC.

## CHILD DEVELOPMENT/DEVELOPMENTAL DELAY: "WHAT YOU DO MATTERS" PARENTING PROGRAM

AAP CATCH Grant/Residents - 2020

Contact: Dana Ribaudo, MD

Wake Forest University School of Medicine, Winston-Salem

## PROGRAM DESCRIPTION

Effective parenting can serve as a buffer for adverse childhood events by minimizing stress and improving overall health. Youth living in socially or economically disadvantaged communities are exposed to higher levels of toxic stress, and are therefore at higher risk for learning delays and decreased kindergarten readiness. Furthermore, children living in households with poverty are more likely to be affected by the social determinants of health. However, unlike many social determinants of health, parenting behaviors are more easily modifiable. Learning effective parenting skills can ultimately lead to parental resilience and improved knowledge of parenting and child development, which can cultivate social and emotional competence in children.

Prevention efforts to combat toxic stress and the social determinants of health have been implemented within the county and at our resident clinic, the Downtown Health Plaza (DHP), one of the largest Medicaid-serving clinics in North Carolina, where 90 percent of patients receive Medicaid, another eight percent are self-pay, and only three percent have private insurance. Examples of prevention efforts include an on-site clinic community partnership with a local early childhood education nonprofit, Imprints Cares. Imprints Cares' mission is to enrich children's development while supporting their families on the journey of parenthood. One of their goals is to impart parenting strategies that will raise more confident, educated, and healthy children. Through on-site clinic programs, broad-based community partnerships, and one-on-one in-home services with family educators, families with children at high risk for developmental delays receive services to foster stronger parenting skills to promote adequate growth and development of their children. Long-term positive impacts of Imprints Cares on the community include higher student achievement and improved behavior, as well as committed and engaged parents. However, while many of our families at the DHP may qualify for home-based visitations, there is a wait list of approximately fifty families for these services.

In recognition of the additional need for parenting support programs for our patients, the purpose of this project is to implement a new parenting skills program for families at the DHP Clinic facilitated by Imprints Cares in conjunction with the Wake Forest Pediatric residency program. This new program will consist of a six-session series developed to support parental knowledge of child development and is designed to be used within a larger family engagement strategy. "What You Do Matters" is an evidence-based parenting curriculum created by Parents as Teachers, the model used by Imprints Cares' home visitation program. Parents as Teachers develops curricula that support a parent's role in promoting school readiness and healthy development of children. Through implementing this new class series with CATCH funding, more families identified by our pediatric residents during continuity clinic visits will benefit from an additional opportunity to learn about healthy child development and network with other families within the community.

Through tracking parent satisfaction, increased parental knowledge, and improved child development, we hope to document program effectiveness that will enable us to secure future funding for expanded parenting skills programs.

**GOALS**

1. Recruit and enroll fifteen high-risk families by August 2020 for the new "What You Do Matters" parenting program in conjunction with Imprints Cares at our resident clinic at the Downtown Health Plaza. By offering incentives, the goal will be for ten high-risk families (66 percent of those recruited) to complete all six sessions of the "What You Do Matters" curriculum by October 2020.

2. Compared to the baseline, families who complete the "What You Do Matters" program by October 2020 will demonstrate a 20 percent improvement in

parent knowledge across three domains, including awareness of performing developmentally appropriate interactions with their children, knowledge of child development, and level of confidence in parenting skills. Additionally, compared to the baseline, children of parents who complete the program will demonstrate a 10 percent improvement in a validated developmental screening tool within three to six months.

3. Families who complete the "What You Do Matters" curriculum will demonstrate an 80 percent satisfaction rate with the program by February 2021.

## WELL-CHILD/WELL-BABY CARE: THE IMMIGRANT LINK

AAP CATCH Grant/Residents – 2021

Contacts: Lisbeth Labrada, MD; Gracen Avis, MD, MPH

Myers Park Pediatrics – Atrium Health Levine Children's Hospital, Charlotte

### PROGRAM DESCRIPTION

Myers Park Pediatrics (MPP) in Charlotte is a general pediatric clinic that serves children of many low-income families and is one of the main education sites for Atrium Health Levine Children's Hospital. As residents, we want to be active participants in creating a medical home for the immigrant children we serve that provides comprehensive, coordinated, and culturally effective care. Our project aims to create a resident-led community engagement team to help link immigrant children and their families with services provided by locally-based organizations. For the purposes of our project, we define immigrant children as foreign-born children whose families speak a primary language other than English. We recognize that this patient population often faces language barriers and specific needs in areas such as mental health, food security, and housing stability. Immigrant children represent one population group of the more than 11,000 unique patients seen at MPP last year; 53 percent of their families were foreign language speaking (45 percent Spanish, 7 percent other), requiring interpreter services. Pediatric residents often meet with these families during clinic encounters but feel under-equipped to provide appropriate community resources to help address some of their needs.

As part of the Atrium Health system, we can access an online Community Resource Hub that lists local relief agencies by zip code. Notably, the current system does not allow for a built-in feedback loop to assess the outcome of referrals. In order to provide the best care possible for our patients, we see a need to assess whether the listed resources meet the needs of immigrant patients and their families. Our resident-led community engagement team will conduct a community assessment and asset mapping, looking for active community organizations that offer services addressing the specific needs of immigrant families. Two pediatric residents,

Lisbeth Labrada and Gracen Davis, will initially create this team and lead the recruitment of future members.

For this project, we aim to create and maintain a current list of relevant community resources easily accessible to residents. We will work extensively with families to connect them with community agencies and to gather information on the accessibility and usefulness of these referrals by conducting interviews with them through the referral process. A goal of our project is to educate and involve other residents in identifying patient needs and initiating referrals. Thus, information derived from family interviews will be used to create realistic education and interactive cases that showcase families' experiences accessing these resources.

These cases will be incorporated into our existing Social Determinants of Health and Global Health resident curriculums. Ultimately, we hope to employ residents to link immigrant families to resources, incorporate lessons learned into a sustainable resident curriculum, and gather data to bring to administration supporting the need for an immigrant patient navigator.

**GOALS**

1. To link immigrant families to community resources and obtain feedback on the outcome of these referrals throughout four months in order to maintain a list of at least twenty updated and relevant community resources.
2. To increase pediatric residents' referrals of immigrant families to appropriate community resources by 50 percent at the completion of the project.
3. To increase pediatric residents' knowledge of the aims and usability of existing community resources that support immigrant families by 75 percent at completion.

# Legislation Referenced in Commentary by Jones and Tayloe

**§ 66-27.1A. Water heater thermostat settings.** (a) The thermostat of any new residential water heater offered for sale or lease for use in a single-family or multifamily dwelling in the State shall be preset by the manufacturer or installer no higher than approximately 120 degrees Fahrenheit (or 49 degrees Celsius). A water heater reservoir temperature may be set higher if it is supplying space heaters that require higher temperatures. For purposes of this section, a water heater shall mean the primary source of hot water for any single-family or multifamily residential dwelling including, but not limited to any solar or other hot water heating systems. (b) Nothing in this section shall prohibit the occupant of a single-family or multiunit residential dwelling with an individual water heater from resetting or having reset the thermostat on the water heater. Any such resetting shall relieve the manufacturer or installer of the water heater and, in the case of a residential dwelling that is leased or rented, also the unit's owner, from liability for damages attributed to the resetting. (c) A warning tag or sticker shall be placed on or near the operating thermostat control of any residential water heater. This tag or sticker shall state that the thermostat settings above the preset temperature may cause severe burns. This tag or sticker may carry such other appropriate warnings as may be agreed upon by manufacturers, installers, and other interested parties. (1991, c. 190, s. 1.)

**§ 14-316. Gun Responsibility Legislation. Current through Session Law 2020-97.** Permitting young children to use dangerous firearms. (a) It shall be unlawful for any person to knowingly permit a child under the age of 12 years to have access to, or possession, custody or use in any manner whatever, of any gun, pistol or other dangerous firearm, whether such weapon be loaded or unloaded, unless the person has the permission of the child's parent or guardian, and the child is under the supervision of an adult. Any person violating the provisions of this section shall be guilty of a Class 2 misdemeanor. (b) Air rifles, air pistols, and BB guns shall not be deemed "dangerous firearms" within the meaning of subsection (a) of this section except in the following counties: Caldwell, Durham, Forsyth, Gaston, Haywood, Mecklenburg, Stokes, Union, Vance.

N.C. Gen. Stat. § 14-316

Amended by 2014 N.C. Sess. Laws 119, s. 10-a, eff. 12/1/2014.Amended by 2013 N.C. Sess. Laws 369, s. 4, eff. 10/1/2013.1913, c. 32; C.S., s. 4441; 1965, c. 813; 1971, c. 309; 1993, c. 539, s. 218; 1994, Ex. Sess., c. 24, s. 14(c).

# The Evolution of Physician-Directed Medicaid

by Greg Adams, MD, FAAP

I have been privileged to experience the honor and joy of practicing pediatrics in the state that I most love. I have had the incredible opportunity to work alongside similar like-minded physicians who care passionately about their patients and the state of health care in NC. My college and medical school years were spent in Ohio, my pediatric residency was completed in Dallas, Texas, and my first few years of practice were in rural Michigan. I was thrilled to be able to return to NC in December of 1986 when I joined pediatricians Dr. Bill Horn, Dr. Bob Ellison, and Dr. Pat Geiger. Bill was the NCPeds representative and encouraged me to join as a member.

During the early days of the formation of Carolina Access, as fourteen regional networks came to compose the starting grounds for Community Care of NC and the Community Care Physicians' Network, I was able to meet several of the leaders. Dr. Steve Wegner, the leader of the AccessCare practices that were part of the Carolina Access network, came to Boone to recruit the pediatricians in our area to become a part of this large statewide network that was mainly comprised of independent rural practices. I began attending the network meetings in Greensboro and was able to work alongside many other great pediatricians from around the state, including Jane Foy, Art Kelly, John Whaley, Steve Edwards, Debbie Ainsworth, Chuck Willson, Betsey Tilson, Christoph Diasio, Graham Barden, Scott St. Clair, Susan Mims, Marian Earls, and Larry Mann, among many others.

The interactions at NCPeds regular meetings fostered a camaraderie and fellowship that enhanced and focused our goals and efforts. Even a duffer like me was welcome on golf outings at the annual meeting. The list of heroes is not complete without noting a few of the many "non-physicians" who have played an incredible role in the growth of both the pediatric society and CCNC/CCPN, such as Tork Wade, Steve Shore, Elizabeth Hudgins, Denise Levis Hewson, and Greg Griggs.

My involvement grew in 2008 when Steve Wegner asked me to be a part of the Multi-Payor Project, which was the forerunner of the Blue Quality Premier Program and dovetailed into the Practice Transformation (PTN) grant to help practices become "medical homes." These efforts necessitated a growing interaction with family medicine physicians such as Chip Watkins. Certainly, family physicians were greatly involved in the origins of CCNC, as exemplified by Allen Dobson's leadership from the beginning. Thus, the emphasis has grown from a Medicaid-only focus to a more complete organization supporting primary care physicians in their practice of high quality, compassionate health care.

Today CCPN has contracts for Medicare Advantage (MA) programs, Blue Premiere of Blue Cross Blue Shield of NC, and a working relationship with the United Health Care's State Health Plan (SHP). We also have working relationships to offer telehealth services (Docsink), communication and billing services (Phreesia), as well as office support (Henry Schein, McKesson, Mag Mutual, and Curi). Soon CCPN will be offering a MEWA (Multiple Employer Welfare Arrangement) plan to assist practices that are looking for an alternative to their expensive insurance plans.

Dedicated doctors have not only nurtured the development of CCNC and the birth of CCPN, they have worked together to improve the delivery of compassionate health care to low-income children and adults. They were instrumental in the creation of NC Health Choice (Child Health Insurance Program) for low-income children who did not qualify for Medicaid. Nearly all of these individuals and their colleagues were, at the same time, highly committed to and involved with NCPeds. While NCPeds was not directly leading the development of CCPN, remaining a "neutral Switzerland" to avoid conflict with any competing interests, the shared goal of improving the care of children in general and specifically caring for low-income and special needs children was a uniting bond. NCPeds' culture and environment were the breeding ground for the communication and cooperation of the many physicians who participated in the statewide effort that has grown into the creation of high-quality primary care medical homes for at least one million low-income patients.

The infrastructure and leadership of NCPeds continue to be real keys to the survival of physician-directed managed care, even in the face of the July 1, 2021, Medicaid Transformation in which five private insurance companies were given the privilege of implementing NC Medicaid!

# History of Community Care of North Carolina

by Greg Adams, MD, FAAP

While North Carolina is widely recognized for its innovative statewide medical home and care management system, few individuals outside of the program understand the evolutionary process by which the state developed this program. Community Care of North Carolina (CCNC) did not rise up as a finished vision; rather, it evolved steadily over twenty-five years, adjusting to changing needs and constantly refining its approach. That cycle of continuous quality improvement continues as CCNC prepares for the new Medicaid system and partnerships with health plans on Medicaid, Medicare, and commercial populations.

**FOUNDING ORGANIZATIONS**

Over this quarter-century, a wide range of organizations has contributed to CCNC's success. Four groups have been involved at every stage of the program's development.

## North Carolina Office of Rural Health and Community Care

Under the leadership of Jim Bernstein, its founder and long-time director, the Office of Rural Health and Community Care (ORHCC) has helped NC's rural and underserved communities develop health services for more than thirty-five years for low-income and vulnerable populations. In addition to a statewide network of Rural Health Centers, ORHCC has worked with the Division of Medical Assistance (NC's Medicaid agency) and other agencies within the NC DHHS to develop community-based approaches to improving care and care outcomes for underserved populations. These efforts have included statewide or regional efforts to improve primary care, behavioral health, long-term care, and hospital and school health services. ORHCC has been responsible for program operations, technical assistance, training, data, and reporting for early development phases in the creation of CCNC.

## North Carolina Division of Medical Assistance (DMA)

NC's Medicaid agency has worked closely with ORHCC to promote and support public, private, state, and community partnerships to improve the quality, efficiency, and cost-effectiveness of care for Medicaid recipients. DMA provided financing and aligned policy and regulation to support the development and operation of CCNC.

## North Carolina Foundation for Advanced Health Programs, Inc.

The Bernstein Foundation (now the Foundation for Health Leadership and Innovation) is a nonprofit established in 1982 to facilitate the development of public-private programs that improve access to efficient and high-quality care for North Carolina's low-income and underserved populations. Since its inception, the Foundation for Health Leadership and Innovation has served as an important catalyst for positive change, promoting public and private state and local development efforts. Much of CCNC's piloting and testing has been sponsored by the Foundation.

## Kate B.Reynolds Charitable Trust

One of North Carolina's oldest and largest health care philanthropies has used its voice and resources to support organizations that address the health needs of the vulnerable, underserved, and economically disadvantaged. At each critical juncture in CCNC's evolution, Kate B. Reynolds (KBR) could be counted on for encouragement and vital seed funds to develop and evaluate key innovations. During the program's early development, KBR provided six grants totaling more than $1.6 million.

**EARLY DEVELOPMENT STEPS PRIOR TO THE LAUNCHING OF CCNC**

## Wilson County Health Plan (1983–1988)

In 1983, NC's Medicaid program was a fee-for-service program that encouraged more physician participation in Medicaid, thereby improving access and reducing recipient reliance on the hospital emergency room. In an effort to evaluate approaches for improving primary care physician participation in Medicaid, the North Carolina Foundation for Advanced Health Programs, in partnership with DMA and ORHCC, submitted a proposal to KBR to pilot NC's first effort at developing medical homes for Medicaid recipients. A KBR grant was received to work with health organizations in Wilson County, a mostly rural county about one hour east of Raleigh.

With a population of approximately 100,000 residents and located in the heart of tobacco country, Wilson County's health infrastructure included two mid-size, multi-specialty group practices, a 250-bed community hospital, a county health department, and a county department of social services. The grant provided funding that enabled these health organizations to work with the state and the Foundation to develop the Wilson County Health Plan.

Under the Wilson County Health Plan, systems and processes were designed and implemented to enable Wilson County Medicaid recipients to enroll with Wilson County's primary care and group practices. These practices agreed to assume responsibility for providing direct services and coordinating enrollee care. A key goal of the project was to reduce the reliance on the hospital emergency room for non-emergency care. The Wilson County Department of Social Services oversaw recipient education and enrollment, while DMA made the changes to the state's eligibility and payment systems that were needed to operate the pilot.

During the implementation, 1,500 Medicaid recipients became members of the Wilson County Health Plan. A first-year evaluation showed a 58 percent decline in emergency room use among enrollees and savings to the state of $300,000. Although the basic operation was considered a great success, a proposed segment of the plan was never implemented. As originally proposed, participating providers would receive a monthly prepaid payment for each enrollee. This proposed payment was designed to cover all outpatient expenses and incent practices to provide more care within the primary care office. Unfortunately, the state's payment system could not accommodate this payment change within the demonstration period.

## Carolina Access (1989–1997)

With the success of the Wilson County Health Plan, KBR approached the Foundation, ORHCC and DMA in 1989 to gauge interest in expanding the medical home model to additional North Carolina counties. The response was immediate and enthusiastic, and KBR agreed to provide a three-year grant to help make it happen.

From 1989 to 1991, the Foundation (in concert with DMA and ORHCC, and with funding from KBR) began expanding the medical home program, which was to become known as Carolina Access, to twelve counties (Beaufort, Burke, Durham, Edgecombe, Greene, Henderson, Madison, Moore, Nash, Pitt, Wayne, and Wilson). While built on the Wilson County Health Plan, the Carolina Access program adopted a new payment mechanism from Kentucky's Ken Pac program. Participating primary care providers would receive $3 per-member per-month payment for each Carolina Access enrollee they served. For this payment, the physician agreed to provide and coordinate an enrollee's care and authorize specialty referrals. As part of this expansion, DMA/ORHCC secured a 1915(b) federal waiver to operate this Primary Care Case Management (PCCM) program and to develop the needed state support and system changes.

With the successful launch of Carolina Access, DMA (with support from the NC General Assembly and the Health Care Financing Administration) began to expand Carolina Access statewide in 1992. By mid-1993, 45,649 Medicaid recipients were enrolled in Carolina Access, and 469 primary care physicians were participating in the program. By the end of 1997, Carolina Access was in place in ninety-nine out of one hundred North Carolina counties (Mecklenburg County remained a managed-care-only county). More than 650,000 Medicaid beneficiaries were enrolled, and more than 2,000 primary care physicians were participating in the program. The Carolina Access program had achieved its primary goals of providing the majority of eligible enrollees (more than 70 percent of women and children recipients were enrolled) with a medical home and in decreasing emergency room visits in non-emergency situations (a reduction of thirty percent).

## Early Days of Community Care of North Carolina (1997–2001)

In the mid-1990s, a number of federal proposals circulating in Washington, DC, called for shifting more of the fiscal responsibility for Medicaid to the states. The Secretary of the NC Department of Health and Human Services asked senior leadership from the Office of Rural Health and DMA to work with the Foundation and other organizations to plan a next-generation Medicaid program that could provide better budget predictability and control. With the assignment came two design directives. First, organizers were asked to build on Carolina Access by creating a medical home model that could improve the quality and cost-effectiveness of care as it improved access. Second, organizers were asked to retain physician support and participation and to achieve lasting improvements in care and care outcomes, focusing design efforts on improving the quality of care rather than seeking quick cuts in program costs. Then-Secretary of Health and Human Services Dr. David Bruton, a pediatrician, was convinced that quality care would be cost-effective care.

In designing the new program, planners worked with state and local medical and government leaders. From this planning effort came the conviction that to improve quality and cost-effectiveness of care, the program must strengthen the medical home by enhancing the ability of the primary care physician to improve care and care outcomes for patients with chronic illnesses through four new program elements:

**The Formation of Networks:** Physicians would be encouraged to work together locally and with other community health organizations that provide direct patient care (e.g., public health departments, hospitals, social services departments, and mental health agencies) to cooperatively plan for meeting recipients' care needs. The primary focus was on recipients with chronic conditions. Chronic illness accounted for a majority of Medicaid expenditures, and the local systems through which these patients received care needed major reform.

**Introduction of Population Management Tools:** To arm the primary care physician and practice with the support and tools to improve care outcomes, the new program would include population management approaches: evidenced-based programs and protocols; disease management programs; care management tools; pharmacy management tools; and practice-based improvements.

**Case Management and Clinical Support:** The new program also would provide the care and case management support needed by physicians to help manage those patients with complex medical, social, and behavioral health conditions who tended to get lost in the existing system.

**Data and Feedback:** Because until this point physicians had limited information on either patient outcomes or progress in improving care, the new program would focus on providing timely and relevant information on how patients and interventions were faring and highlighting opportunities for improvement.

After the Secretary endorsed the draft plan in 1997, a statewide meeting was convened with health and civic leaders to discuss the plan, solicit feedback, and secure support for conducting a pilot. There was nearly unanimous support for the approach. The next step was to gauge the level of interest of key physicians participating in the Carolina Access program. In early 1998, the Secretary asked all Carolina Access practices with at least 2,000 enrollees (36 practices) to indicate their interest in partnering with the state. The response was overwhelming—all but one practice wanted to participate. Practices were given two options. They could work together as physician groups and form a horizontal network that would cross many communities; or they could join with other local practices and health organizations to form a community network.

Twenty-six practices, almost all of them pediatric, applied to work together to form a statewide physician's network. Nine practices wanted to form community networks (Pitt, Durham, Surry, Guilford, Cabarrus, Buncombe, Gaston, and Cleveland counties). Each of these new networks represented a different lead provider (private physician groups, Academic Health Center, Health Department, FQHC, PHO), but all formed under a similar principle of being not-for-profit and collaborative.

In early 1998, the state received approval from the Health Care Financing Administration to amend its 1915(b) federal waiver to develop the successor program to Carolina Access, which initially was known as Carolina Access II and Access III. With federal approval secured, the new program began as a pilot in July of that year.

## THE OFFICIAL LAUNCH OF COMMUNITY CARE OF NORTH CAROLINA (2001–2020)

January 2001 marked the beginning of a new administration for NC and DHHS, as incoming Governor Mike Easley appointed Carmen Hooker Odom Secretary of Health and Human Services. Secretary Hooker Odom asked Jim Bernstein, the long-time leader of the ORHCC, to join her as Assistant Secretary of Health and Human Services. The first year saw major budget pressure on Medicaid because of a state economic downturn. While there were excellent early results in quality improvement and cost savings with the Access II and III program, the program involved only ten counties plus the large pediatric network, far from a statewide program.

After a careful review, Secretary Hooker Odom determined that Access II and III should be expanded statewide as the major initiative to manage Medicaid cost and quality, and renamed the program Community Care of North Carolina (CCNC). The next four years saw the expansion of local networks to adjoining counties, and the organization of new networks covering the majority of North Carolina. As of May 2011, fourteen CCNC networks cover all one hundred counties in the state, serving more than one million enrollees (1,000,024 Medicaid recipients and 70,000 low-income uninsured residents through the HealthNet Program).

In 2005, Dr. Allen Dobson, an early leader of CCNC, succeeded Jim Bernstein as Assistant Secretary of Health and Human Services and the state's Medicaid Director. Although CCNC had achieved satisfactory results in managing the Aid to Families with Dependent Children (AFDC) population, the Medicaid budget still experienced high yearly cost growth. Dr. Dobson asked CCNC to begin to manage the costliest Medicaid recipients, e.g., the aged, blind, and disabled. The NC General Assembly appropriated $6 million of state funds for the program to extend its community-based model to aged, blind, and disabled recipients. After two years of intense work on this pilot, the major chronic care initiative was rolled out program wide with excellent results.

Late in 2005, Secretary Hooker-Odom, Dr. Dobson, Torlen Wade, the head of the ORHCC and early leader of CCNC, and Dr. Bill Roper, dean of the UNC School of Medicine and former administrator of the Health Care Financing Administration, presented to Centers for Medicare and Medicaid Services (CMS) Administrator

Mark McClellan a plan to extend CCNC's role to the management of recipients dually eligible for Medicare and Medicaid and at-risk Medicare recipients. This group proposed a shared savings demonstration with Medicare and led to the formation of a central organization representing all fourteen CCNC networks to apply to the CMS for the demonstration project.

Through its new central organization, CCNC, in late 2006, applied to the CMS to participate in a five-year Medicare Quality Demonstration (646) to "improve the quality of care and service delivered to Medicare beneficiaries through major system redesign." Under this demonstration, CCNC managed approximately 44,000 dually eligible beneficiaries in the first two years. At the beginning of the third year, an estimated 173,808 Medicare-only beneficiaries were added to the demonstration.

In 2006, the Governor's health policy staff and DHHS began work on a statewide public-private quality initiative that brought together the state's largest insurers (Blue Cross and Blue Shield of North Carolina, the State Employee Health Plan, and Medicaid) and providers (the North Carolina Medical Society, North Carolina Pediatric Society, North Carolina Academy of Family Physicians, and University of North Carolina School of Medicine) to collaboratively develop and implement a common set of best medical quality standards and measures for five diseases and/ or conditions (asthma, diabetes, congestive heart failure, hypertension, and post-myocardial infarction care). All participants agreed to implement the Governor's Quality Initiative through the CCNC system. The initiative was launched in 2008.

In 2007, CCNC received the prestigious Annie E. Casey Innovations in American Government Award from the Ash Institute at the Kennedy School of Government at Harvard University for its work in improving health care services for Medicaid and other populations.

In late 2007, a decision was made to gradually transfer much of the responsibility of additional CCNC program development and support from the state to the new central not-for-profit organization representing all fourteen CCNC networks. This would allow for the development of a robust informatics support system to help networks manage recipients and to provide for stability of leadership as CCNC became the key Foundation for many of the state's health care initiatives. Many of the early CCNC leaders are still actively involved in this important program: Drs. Dobson, Bruton, Jones, Wegner, Willson, Earl, Tilson, Ponzi, and Clements, along with Torlen Wade and Denise Levis-Hewson, among others. As health care reform discussions have sparked much activity across the country, CCNC remains a foundational element in much of the work in NC to achieve improved quality at lower costs. These efforts have been estimated to save millions of dollars each year, as calculated by external evaluations. A June 2011 analysis from Treo Solutions found that CCNC saved nearly $1.5 billion in 2007, 2008, and 2009 alone. A December

2011 analysis by Milliman, a national consulting firm based in California, found that CCNC saved the State of North Carolina nearly a billion dollars over a four-year period from 2007 through 2010. A report issued in 2015 by the North Carolina State Auditor estimated CCNC savings at nine percent, working out to approximately a three to one net return on investment in CCNC for the Medicaid program.

In 2016, Hearst Health and the Jefferson College of Population Health of Thomas Jefferson University named CCNC the winner of the inaugural Hearst Health Prize, a $100,000 award given in recognition of outstanding achievement in managing or improving health. CCNC was recognized for its model for managing transitional care for North Carolina Medicaid beneficiaries discharged home after hospitalization.

## CCNC'S TRANSITION TO MANAGED CARE (2020 AND BEYOND)

Beginning with legislation passed in the fall of 2015, North Carolina began preparations to shift to a statewide managed care system for running its Medicaid program. The state released a request for proposal (RFP) for Prepaid Health Plans (PHPs) in the fall of 2018. This resulted in five PHPs being selected to manage the state's Medicaid program, with a portion of the state's Medicaid population remaining in the existing fee-for-service program. Portions of this population will later be transitioned into the managed care program at a later date.

The Department was on track to go live February 1, 2020; however, new funding and program authority were required from the NC General Assembly to meet this timeline, and Medicaid Managed Care was temporarily suspended. Medicaid Managed Care was then scheduled to go live on July 1, 2021.

CCNC responded to this new environment by significantly upgrading and restructuring its core business and quality improvement functions. The Medicaid responsibilities of a number of previously independent 501(c)(3) networks were transferred to CCNC, along with a significant increase in full-time CCNC, Inc. staff to manage this workload. Job descriptions, workflow processes, and for-practice management and care management were standardized, streamlined, and supported with improved analytics and new technical tools. A statewide system combining regional care management and practice support operations now provides a seamless infrastructure across North Carolina.

At the same time, CCNC and Community Care Physician Network, LLC, a clinically integrated network of primary care clinicians, entered into agreements with all five Prepaid Health Plans awarded Medicaid contracts by the state. The contracts vary somewhat in terms of structure and geographic reach, but in all, the aim has been to reduce the administrative load on physicians participating in Medicaid by providing a more uniform approach to care management and quality improvement across all participating PHP populations.

**LEADERSHIP CHANGES**

In January 2021, Dr. Dobson, CCNC's founding president/CEO, retired, and Tom Wroth, MD, MPH, was appointed by the CCNC Board of Directors to replace him.

Dr. Wroth now serves as president/CEO of Community Care of North Carolina, Inc. He is a practicing family physician who has cared for patients for more than twenty years in Alamance and Caswell counties. He is the former chief medical officer at Piedmont Health, a system of ten FQHCs and two PACE sites. Dr. Wroth trained in Family Medicine and Preventive Medicine at UNC–Chapel Hill, and was previously on faculty there in the Department of Family Medicine. He attended medical school at Columbia University, College of Physicians and Surgeons.

Under Dr. Wroth's leadership, CCNC is playing a major role in assisting North Carolina in managing the pandemic, including a partnership with NC Area Health Education centers aimed at helping providers understand and cope with COVID-19 programs to boost rates of childhood immunization that have fallen since the pandemic began, as well as regular webinars and communications keeping providers up-to-date with the latest COVID-19 developments and Medicaid policy changes. In addition, Dr. Wroth has made a company-wide commitment to Diversity, Access, Equity, and Inclusion a top priority for the organization.

# Severe Combined Immunodeficiency (SCID)

By John Meidl, NCPeds, June 3, 2015

SCID, also known as the "bubble boy" disease, is treatable with a bone marrow transplant when caught early. Treatment during the first three and a half months of life greatly increases the chance of survival (93 percent compared to 69 percent), and the efficacy of treatment is much higher for SCID than for most of the metabolic diseases for which we screen. Untreated, the condition is fatal before the first birthday.

Screening for SCID is best practice. It is recommended by the Secretary's Advisory Committee on Heritable Disorders of Infants and Children, US Secretary of HHS, and NC Newborn Screening Committee. Twenty-nine states screen for SCID.

The incidence of SCID is higher than initially thought. Earlier estimates were that about one out of every 100,000 newborns had SCID. However, a recent analysis published in the *Journal of the American Medical Association* found the incidence to be 1:58,000. (Experts suggest that many infant deaths were previously attributed to pneumonia or other infections before a diagnosis of SCID was established.) North Carolina has approximately 120,000 to 130,000 births each year.

NC has a low newborn screening fee at $19, the sixth lowest in the nation. Surrounding states have fees at least twice as much: SC $68.51, TN $75, and VA

$53. The cost of treating SCID for healthy babies is about one-twentieth the cost of performing a transplant for sicker SCID babies due to the cost of treating their infections. Diagnosing SCID at birth allows the transplant to be performed before infections are acquired due to the infant's absent immune system.

In the House Health Committee hearing on May 20, 2015, Dr. Becky Buckley, Professor of Pediatrics and Immunology at Duke University Medical Center, which has done more SCID transplants than any single center in the world and has one of the highest survival rates, testified the cost of treatment is about $100,000 for a healthy SCID infant. In contrast, the four NC babies she has transplanted over the past five years, all of whom were diagnosed late and were extremely sick, incurred costs totaling $14 million. (Of that sum, $10 million was charged to Medicaid and $4 million to private insurance.)

The Baby Carlie Nugent Bill (H698) adds SCID to the required panel of newborn screening. It uses $466,000 in funding from the House Budget (H97) to match a federal grant (HRSA) for a one-time purchase of equipment and related programming and training. It increases the newborn screening fee from $19 to $24 to cover the marginal cost of the screen. It passed the House with a vote of 109-1 in September 2015.

## Kids in Parks

Kids in Parks (KIP) adventures are designed to get children and their families outdoors to practice active living. Drs. Olson Huff and Bob Schwartz, concerned about the sedentary lifestyles of children and increases in the incidence of overweight and obesity, promoted the idea of using trails on the Blue Ridge Parkway (BRP). The Superintendent of the BRP and The Blue Ridge Parkway Foundation enthusiastically agreed, and the first trail was opened in 2008 at Parkway Headquarters, Asheville. The Blue Cross and Blue Shield of North Carolina Foundation gave funds to initiate and sustain the program.

KIP is now in fourteen states and the District of Columbia, with more than 250 adventure trails to encourage healthy activity and learning about the natural environment. Each trailhead features a description of animal and plant life that hikers may encounter. Trails are chosen for safety and to accommodate children with health and physical challenges so that no child misses an opportunity to enjoy the outdoors. Pediatricians are encouraged to write a prescription for a hike. Visit kidsinparks.com to learn more and find an adventure.

# NCPeds Awards
# 1987-2022

# NCPeds Awards 1987-2022

**DAVID T. TAYLOE SR. AWARD FOR OUTSTANDING COMMUNITY SERVICE**

Given to a pediatrician who has made exceptional contributions in her/his local community or statewide, and what may include efforts beyond the practice setting.

## Past Recipients

2022 David L. Hill, MD, FAAP, Goldsboro

2021 Rasheeda Monroe, MD, FAAP, Raleigh

2020 Laura Gerald, MD, MPH, FAAP, Raleigh

2019 John W. Rusher, JD, MD, FAAP, Raleigh

2018 Gerri Mattson, MD, MPH, FAAP, Chapel Hill

2017 Julie Linton, MD, FAAP, Winston-Salem

2016 Graham Barden III, MD, FAAP, New Bern

2016 Christoph Diasio, MD, FAAP, Southern Pines

2015 Jane Meschan Foy, MD, FAAP, Oak Ridge

2014 Robert "Rip" V. Ford, MD, Winston-Salem

2013 Charles Scott, MD, Burlington

2012 Tamara Coyne-Beasley, MD, Durham

2011 Marian F. Earls, MD, Greensboro

2010 Jerry C. Bernstein, MD, Raleigh

2009 Sue Hollowell Lee, MD, Bayboro

2008 Joseph T. Bell, MD, Lumberton

2007 Deborah L. Ainsworth, MD, Washington

2006 Steve Wegner, MD, JD, Chapel Hill

2005 John G. Johnston, MD, Charlotte

2004 Joseph W. Ponzi, MD, Goldsboro

2003 Frederick D. Burroughs, MD, Raleigh

2002 Olson Huff, MD, Black Mountain

2001 C. Lee Gilliatt Jr., MD, Shelby

2000 Robert L. Young, MD, Lumberton

1999 Wallace D. Brown, MD, Raleigh

1998 Peter J. Morris, MD, Fuquay-Varina

1997 Charles L. Kennedy, MD, Winston-Salem

1996 David T. Tayloe Jr., MD, Goldsboro

1995 William R. Purcell, MD, Laurinburg

1994 David R. Williams Sr., MD, Thomasville

1993 H. David Bruton, MD, Southern Pines

1992 Jonnie Horn McLeod, MD, Charlotte

1991 Andrea Gravatt, MD, Asheville

**DENNY, KATZ, SIMON, TINGELSTAD ACADEMIC SERVICE AWARD**

Given to an academic pediatrician member for outstanding efforts to improve the health and wellness of all children in North Carolina.

## Past Recipients

2022 Kathleen Bartlett, MD, Durham
2022 Meg Kihlstrom, MD, FAAP, Chapel Hill
2022 Sarah Leondar, MD, MPH, Greenville
2022 Mia Mallory, MD, Durham
2022 Kenya McNeal-Trice, MD, FAAP, Chapel Hill
2022 Sydney Primis, MD, FAAP, Charlotte
2022 Thomas Russell, MD, Charlotte
2022 Betty Staples, MD
2019 Coleen Cunningham, MD, FAAP, Raleigh
2018 Eliana M. Perrin, MD, MPH, FAAP, Chapel Hill
2017 Amina Ahmed, MD, FAAP, FPIDS, Charlotte
2016 Charles F. Willson, MD, FAAP, Farmville
2015 Julie Story Byerley, MD, FAAP, Chapel Hill
2014 Jacob A. Lohr, MD, FAAP, Chapel Hill
2013 Dale A. Newton, MD, FAAP, Greenville
2012 J. Edward Spence, MD, FAAP, Charlotte
2011 David Ingram, MD, FAAP, Raleigh
2010 Harvey J. Hamrick, MD, FAAP, Chapel Hill
2010 Sarah Hendricks Sinal, MD, FAAP, Winston-Salem
2009 Kenneth B. Roberts, MD, FAAP, Greensboro
2008 Jon S. Abramson, MD, FAAP, Winston-Salem
2007 Alan D. Stiles, MD, FAAP, Chapel Hill
2006 Dennis A Clements III, MD, MPH, PhD, FAAP, Durham
2005 Jane Meschan Foy, MD, FAAP, Oak Ridge
2004 Karen Hillenbrand, MD, FAAP, Greenville
2003 V. Denise Everett, MD, FAAP, Raleigh
2002 Robert P. Schwartz, MD, FAAP, Winston-Salem

**AWARD FOR OUTSTANDING ACHIEVEMENT**

Given to a pediatrician or professional working in pediatrics who has given exceptional service to improve the health and well-being of infants, children, adolescents, and young adults.

## Past Recipients

2017 Brandy Bynum Dawson, MPA, Raleigh
2013 Gerri Mattson, MD, MPH, FAAP, Chapel Hill
2012 Jimmy L. Simon, MD, FAAP, Winston-Salem
2011 Sarah C. Armstrong, MD, FAAP, Durham
2009 William W. Lawrence Jr., MD, FAAP, Durham
2009 K. Michael Dennis, MD, FAAP, Hendersonville
2008 Rebecca R. Socolar, MD, MPH, FAAP, Durham
2008 Robert P. Schwartz, MD, FAAP, Winston-Salem

**AWARD FOR OUTSTANDING ACHIEVEMENT, *CONTINUED***

2007 Elwood B. Coley, MD, FAAP, Lumberton
2006 Samuel L. Katz, MD, FAAP, Durham
2003 C. Ellis Fisher, MD, FAAP, Gastonia
2002 George A. Engstrom, MD, FAAP, Concord
2000 Thomas Vitaglione, MPH, Raleigh

## GOOD FOR KIDS AWARD

Given to an individual or organization that initiates or participates in a community or statewide effort to improve the quality of life for infants, children, adolescents, or young adults.

## Past Recipients

2018 Joseph A. Ponzi, JD, Greensboro,
   Partner, Brooks, Pierce, McLendon, Humphrey & Leonard, LLP
2016 Alamance Partnership for Children (Smart Start), Burlington
2015 Anita Farel, DrPH, Chapel Hill, UNC Gillings School of Public Health,
   Maternal and Child Health
2015 Jesse Lewis, Peacemakers of Rocky Mount
2013 North Carolina Infant and Young Child Mental Health Association
2012 The Governor Morehead School for the Blind, Raleigh
2012 Prevent Blindness North Carolina, Jennifer Talbot, Executive Director, Raleigh
2012 Governor's Vision Commission, Ophthalmologist Members: Michael Bartiss, OD, MD,
   Southern Pines; David Wallace, MD, MPH, FAAO, Durham; William Young, MD, FAAP, FAAO,
   Greensboro; Peter J. Morris, MD, MPH, MDiv, FAAP, Fuquay-Varina
2011 Cameron Graham, MPH, Raleigh
2010 The NC Health & Wellness Trust Fund Commission, Raleigh
2009 Jeffrey Simms, MSPH, MDiv, Raleigh, NC Division of Medical Assistance
2009 Carolyn Sexton, BSN, MPH, Raleigh, NC Division of Public Health
2009 Holy Angels, Services for the Differently Able, Belmont
2008 Pamela Seamans, MPP, Executive Director, NC Alliance for Health
2008 Kathleen Clarke-Pearson, MD, FAAP, Southern Pines
2008 Brian Lewis, MPA, Executive Director, Covenant with NC's Children
2008 William Taub, MSW, Durham, Director, Duke's Camp Kaleidoscope
2007 Kelly Haupt, RDH, MPA, Raleigh, NC's Oral Health Dental Varnish Program,
   "Into the Mouths of Babes"
2007 Patricia Garrett, PhD, Raleigh, Director, Covering Kids and Families
2007 Sue L. Makey, CAE, Newton Grove, Executive Vice President, NC Academy of Family Physicians
2007 Joyce Moore, RN, FNE, MPH, Chapel Hill, NC's Child Medical Evaluation Program
2006 Dr. Luanne K. Williams, Raleigh, State Epidemiologist, Occupational & Environmental
   Epidemiology Branch, NC Division of Public Health
2006 Kelly Ransdell, Raleigh, State Coordinator, Safe Kids North Carolina,
   NC Department of Insurance, East Carolina University/University Health Services,
   Pediatric Health Weight Research and Treatment Center
2006 Diane Lewis Sloane, Raleigh, Program Coordinator, NC Pediatric Society
2005 The Agriculture Resources Center, Carrboro, Alan Spalt, Executive Director

**GOOD FOR KIDS AWARD,** *CONTINUED*

2005 The North Carolina Child Advocacy Institute, Raleigh, Barbara Bradley, Executive Director
2003 Sari Teplin, MPH, Chapel Hill, Covering Kids Director
2001 June Milby, Raleigh, NC Division of Medical Assistance, NC Health Choice Coordinator
2000 Stephanie Fanjul, Raleigh, Smart Start Executive Director, Childcare Star-Rated Licensure
1999 Adrian Sandler, MD, Asheville, Buncombe County Gun Safety Project
1999 Ellen Roberts, RN, MPH, Greensboro, Reach Out and Read
1998 Paula Wolf, Raleigh, Covenant with NC's Children
1998 Thomas J. Dimmock, Raleigh, "Pull the Plug on Media Violence"
1998 Frank Herbert, Asheville, Generous Support to NCPeds Programs

**JAMES D. BERNSTEIN EXCELLENCE IN PUBLIC SERVICE TO CHILDREN AWARD**
Originally called the Legislative Award; renamed the Excellence in Public Service to Children Award; now named in honor of James D. Bernstein, founder and director of the NC Office of Rural Health.

Given to a public servant in either the executive or legislative branch of government in recognition of outstanding achievement to improve the health and well-being of infants, children, adolescents, and young adults.

### Legislative Award

1991 NC Representative David Diamont, Pilot Mountain
1990 NC House Representative Theresa Esposito, Winston-Salem
1990 NC House Representative Narvel Jim Crawford, Asheville
1989 NC Senator James Ezzell Jr., Rocky Mount
1989 NC Senator Helen Marvin, Gastonia
1989 NC House Representative Joe Hackney, Chapel Hill
1988 NC Senator Russell Walker, Asheboro
1988 NC House Representative Ruth Easterling, Charlotte
1987 NC House Representative Marie Colton, Asheville
1987 NC Senator Charles Hipps, Waynesville

### Excellence in Public Service to Children Award

2004 NC Representative Edd Nye, Bladenboro
2003 NC Representative Martin Nesbitt, Asheville
2002 NC Senator William R. Purcell, MD, FAAP, Laurinburg
2001 H. David Bruton, MD, Southern Pines, Secretary, NC Department of Health and Human Services
2000 Paul R. (Dick) Perruzi, Director, NC Division of Medical Assistance, Raleigh
1999 NC House Representative Phillip S. Baddour, Jr., Goldsboro
1998 Lieutenant Governor Dennis Wicker, Sanford, State of North Carolina, Raleigh
1997 Attorney General Michael F. Easley, Southport, State of North Carolina, Raleigh
1996 Margaret Arbuckle, MEd. PhD, Greensboro, Chairperson, NC Child Advocacy Institute, Raleigh
1995 Dennis Williams, NC Division of Medical Assistance, Raleigh
1994 Ann F. Wolfe, MD, FAAP, NC Division of Public Health, Raleigh
1994 Governor James B. Hunt Jr., State of North Carolina, Raleigh
1993 Barbara Matula, Director, NC Division of Medical Assistance, Raleigh
1993 NC House Representative Dub Dickson, Gastonia

**EXCELLENCE IN PUBLIC SERVICE TO CHILDREN AWARD,** *CONTINUED*

1992 Henry Jones Jr., JD, NCPeds Lobbyist, Raleigh
1992 Tom Vitaglione, MPH, NC Division of Public Health, Raleigh

## *James D. Bernstein Excellence in Public Service to Children Award*

2022 Theresa M. Flynn, MD, MPH, FAAP, WakeMed Physicians, Raleigh
2021 Shannon Dowler, MD, FAAFP, Chief Medical Officer, NC Medicaid,
   NC Department of Health and Human Services, Raleigh
2020 Mandy Cohen, MD, Secretary, NC Department of Health and Human Services, Raleigh
2019 Dave Richard, Deputy Secretary for Medicaid,
   NC Department of Health and Human Services, Raleigh
2018 Gregory F. Murphy, MD, US House of Representatives, Member of Congress, Greenville
2017 Megan Davies, MD, State Epidemiologist, Chief of the NC Epidemiology Section,
   NC Division of Public Health, Raleigh
2015 Josephine Cialone, MS, RD, Supplemental Nutrition Program for Women,
   Infants and Children (WIC), NC Division of Public Health, Raleigh
2015 Sandy Terrell, MS, RN, NC Division of Medical Assistance, Raleigh
2014 Kevin Ryan, MD, MPH, NC Division of Public Health, Raleigh
2013 Tara R. Larson, Division of Medical Assistance; NC Division of Mental Health,
   Developmental Disabilities & Substance Abuse Services, Washington, NC
2012 Attorney General Roy A. Cooper III, State of North Carolina, Raleigh
2011 Torlen (Tork) Wade, MPH,Community Care of North Carolina, Raleigh
2010 Chris G. Hoke, JD, Chief of Regulatory and Legal Affairs, NC Division of Public Health, Raleigh
2009 Leah McCall Devlin, DDS, MPH, North Carolina State Health Director, Raleigh
2008 NC House Representative Jeffrey Barnhart, Concord
2008 NC House Representative Jennifer Weiss, Cary
2007 NC House Representative Martha Bedell Alexander, Charlotte
2007 NC House Representative Verla C. Insko, Chapel Hill
2006 Lieutenant Governor Beverly Eaves Perdue, New Bern, State of North Carolina, Raleigh
2005 James D. Bernstein, MPH, Chapel Hill, Director, NC Office of Rural Health, Raleigh
2005 Beth Rowe-West, RN, BSN, Thomasville, Chief, NC Immunization Branch,
   NC Division of Public Health, Raleigh

## RISING STAR EARLY CAREER PHYSICIAN AWARD

Given to a pediatrician within their first ten years of completion of post-graduate training, in residency or fellowship, who has demonstrated excellence in the community by contributions to clinical medicine, research, education, or advocacy in Pediatrics.

2019 Gabriela Maradiaga Panayotti, MD
2018 Emily B. Vander Schaff, MD, MPH, FAAP
2017 Yun Boylston, MD, FAAP

**HONORARY MEMBERSHIP AWARD**

Given to a pediatrician member who has an accomplished career of outstanding work in the field of pediatrics and made substantial contributions to NCPeds activities, advocacy and accomplishments.

## Past Recipients

Jay Arena, Durham

Wallace D. (Wally) Brown, Raleigh

H. David Bruton, Southern Pines

Susan Dees, Durham

Floyd W. Denny Jr., Chapel Hill

E. Stephen Edwards, Raleigh

George A. Engstrom, Concord

William W. Farley, Raleigh

Thomas Eliot Frothingham, Durham

Charles Gay, Charlotte

Kenneth Geddie, High Point

William (Bill) C. Hubbard, Raleigh

Olson Huff, Black Mountain

Henry W. Johnson, Winston-Salem

Samuel L. Katz, Durham

Charlie L. Kennedy, Winston-Salem

William Lord London, Durham

John F. Lynch Jr., High Point

Angus M. McBryde, Durham

Jonnie Horn McLeod, Charlotte

James C. Parke Jr., Charlotte

George E. Prince, Gastonia

Fletcher Raiford, Hendersonville

Frank R. Reynolds, Wilmington

Jimmie L. Rhyne, Raleigh

Oliver F. Roddey Jr., Charlotte

Robert P. Schwartz, Winston-Salem

Jimmy L. Simon, Winston-Salem

David T. Tayloe Sr., Washington

Jon B. Tingelstad, Chocowinity

G. Earl Trevathan, Greenville

Bailey Webb, Durham

Thad B. Wester, Lumberton

David R. Williams Sr., Thomasville

**STEVE SHORE SERVICE AWARD**

Given to an individual or organization that has demonstrated unwavering interest in, and loyalty to, NCPeds for a minimum of five years. Particular consideration is given to members who have taken the initiative to serve effectively on behalf of NCPeds and who have responded to requests for service to assist NCPeds (not a requirement). Formerly called the Award of Appreciation for service to NCPeds, re-named to honor Steve Shore, executive director of NCPeds (1999-2014).

## Past Recipients

2019 Norma Marti, BA, Raleigh, Minority Outreach Consultant,
    NC Department of Health & Human Services
2018 David L. Hill, MD, FAAP, Goldsboro
2017 John W. Rusher, JD, MD, FAAP, Raleigh
2016 Kenya McNeal-Trice, MD, FAAP, Chapel Hill
2015 Elizabeth Cuervo Tilson, MD, MPH, FAAP, Raleigh
2014 Steve Shore, MSW, Apex
2011 W. Scott St. Clair, MD, FAAP, Boone
2010 Judy Wood, MD, Greenville
2010 Gregg Talente, MD, Columbia, SC
2008 Julie Story Byerley, MD, MPH, Chapel Hill
2008 W. Scott St. Clair, MD, FAAP, Boone
2008 Andrew R. Shulstad, MD, FAAP, Charlotte
2005 Sharon McGarry Foster, MD, FAAP, Raleigh
2001 Tracey Bradshaw, Winston-Salem, Wake Forest University School of Medicine,
    Department of Pediatrics
2001 Marcia E. Herman-Giddens, PA, MPH, DrPH, Chapel Hill,
    UNC Gillings School of Public Health

**TOM VITAGLIONE CHILD HEALTH ADVOCACY AWARD**

Given to an individual or organization from the nonprofit sector for outstanding achievement or advocacy efforts.

## Past Recipients

2019 Kathleen Clarke-Pearson, MD, FAAP, Chapel Hill
2018 Legal Aid of North Carolina
2017 Beth Messersmith, MPA, Durham
2015 Greg Griggs, MPA, CAE, Henderson
2015 Karen McLeod, MSW, Raleigh
2014 Karen St. Clair, MD, FAAP, Durham
2013 Elizabeth Hudgins, MPP, Raleigh
2012 Michelle Hughes, MSW, Raleigh
2011 Steve Shore, MSW, Apex
2010 Barbara Bradley, Raleigh
2009 Pam Silberman, JD, DrPH, Chapel Hill
2008 Tom Vitaglione, MPH, Raleigh
2008 Adam Searing, JD, MPH, Chapel Hill

# Contributors

# List of Contributors

**Greg Adams, MD, FAAP**
Co-President, Community Care Physician Network, Raleigh
Chief of Pediatrics, Community Care of North Carolina, Raleigh
Founder of Blue Ridge Pediatrics, Boone (Retired)

**Amina Ahmed, MD, FAAP, FPIDS**
Medical Director of Pediatric Infectious Disease and Immunology, Hospital Epidemiologist,
    Atrium Health Levine Children's Hospital, Charlotte, NC
Past member, NC Committees on Infectious Diseases, Vaccines and Immunizations

**Deborah Ainsworth, MD, FAAP**
Pediatrician, Washington Pediatrics, Washington, NC
Past President, NCPeds

**Joseph Bell, MD, FAAP (Lumbee)**
Medical Director and Senior Pediatrician, Children's Health Pembroke, Pembroke, NC
Pediatrician, Catawba Indian Health Service Unit, Rock Hill, SC
Member and Past President, Association of American Indian Physicians (AAIP)
AAIP Liaison to AAP Committee on Native American Child Health
Board, NC American Indian Health Board

**Molly Curtin Berkoff, MD, MPH**
Medical Director, NC Child Medical Evaluation Program
Section Head, Child Maltreatment
Professor, Department of Pediatrics, Division of General Pediatrics,
    University of North Carolina School of Medicine
Public Health Pediatrician, Wake County Health and Human Services, Raleigh, NC

**Debra Best, MD, FAAP**
Associate Professor of Pediatrics, Division of General Pediatrics and Adolescent Health,
    Duke University School of Medicine
Co-Associate Director, AAP Community Pediatrics Training Initiative (CPTI)
NC Chair, CPTI Carolinas Collaborative

**Thomas F. Boat, MD, FAAP**
Professor of Pediatrics, Cincinnati Children's Hospital Medical Center and University of Cincinnati
Former Dean, University of Cincinnati College of Medicine (2010-14)
Former Chair, Department of Pediatrics, UNC (1982-93) and University of Cincinnati (1993-2007)

**Yun Boylston, MD, MBA, FAAP**
Pediatrician, Burlington Pediatrics and Mebane Pediatrics
Board member, NCPeds

**Julie Story Byerley, MD, MPH**
President and Dean, Geisinger Commonwealth School of Medicine
Executive VP and Chief Academic Officer, Geisinger
Former Residency Program Director, Vice Dean for Education, UNC School of Medicine

**Kathleen Clarke-Pearson, MD, FAAP**
(see *Acknowledgements: NCPeds Steering Committee*)

**Herb Clegg, MD, FAAP**
Pediatrician, Novant Health Eastover Pediatrics (1982-2015)
Pediatric ID Consultant, Novant Health Hemby Children's Hospital and Atrium Levine Children's
    Hospital (1982-2019)
Senior Vice President for Clinical Excellence, Novant Health (2012-19)
President, Novant Health Medical Group (2008-12)
Past President, NCPeds
Clinical Consultant, Health Resources & Services Administration (2020-present)

**Mandy K. Cohen, MD, MPH**
Secretary, NC Department of Health and Human Services (2017-21)
Chief Executive Officer, Aledade Care Solutions (2022-23)
Director, Centers for Disease Control (2023-present)

**Stephanie Duggins Davis, MD**
Edward C. Curnen Jr. Distinguished Professor & Chair of Pediatrics, UNC School of Medicine
Physician-in-Chief, UNC Children's - NC Children's Hospital
Former Chair, Board of Directors, American Board of Pediatrics
Elected member, American Pediatric Society
Former President, Society of Pediatric Research

**Christoph Diasio, MD, FAAP**
Pediatrician, Sandhills Pediatrics, Southern Pines, NC
Co-Chair, NC Pediatric Council
AAP Vision 2020 Task Force
AAP Section on Pediatric Management (Chair 2014-18)
Past President, NCPeds

**Allen Dobson Jr., MD, FAAFP**
Family Physician and Founding Partner, Cabarrus Family Medicine
Founding Residency Director, Cabarrus Family Medicine Residency Program
Past President, NC Academy of Family Physicians
Assistant Secretary of NC DHHS and Medicaid Director (2005-08)
Past President and CEO, Community Care of NC
Editor in Chief, Medical Economics

**Judith C. Dolins, MPH**
Former Chief Implementation Officer and Senior Vice President, Community and Chapter Affairs
    and Quality Improvement, American Academy of Pediatrics
Title V Lifetime Achievement Award (2020)

**Shannon Dowler, MD, FAAFP**
Chief Medical Officer, NC Medicaid
Assistant Secretary Health Access, NC Department of Health and Human Services
Past President, NC Academy of Family Physicians

**Marian Earls, MD, MTS, FAAP**
Developmental-Behavioral Pediatrician, NICU Developmental Follow-up Clinic,
    Cone Health, Greensboro (1988-present)
Director, Pediatric Programs and Deputy Chief Medical Officer, Community Care of NC (2012-19)
Leader, NC CHIPRA Quality Demonstration Grant (2010-15)
Medical Director, Guilford Child Health (1994-2012)
Director, NC Assuring Better Child Health and Development Program (1999-2019)
Past President, NC Peds
Founder, NCPeds Fostering Health NC Project
Chair, AAP Council on Healthy Mental and Emotional Development (2022-present)
Past Chair, AAP Mental Health Leadership Workgroup (2014-22)
Past Executive Committee member, AAP Council on Early Childhood (2013-17)
AAP Liaison to the American Academy of Child and Adolescent Psychiatry,
    Collaborative and Integrated Care Committee
Board Member, National Network of Child Psychiatry Access Programs

**Beverly Edwards, MD, FAAP**
Lead Pediatrician, Ahoskie Pediatrics, Ahoskie, NC

**E. Stephen (Steve) Edwards, MD, FAAP**
(see *Acknowledgements: NCPeds Steering Committee*)

**V. Denise Everett, MD, FAAP**
Deputy Medical Director, NC Medicaid Management Information System NCTracks Account
CSRA State and Local Solutions, LLC,
    A General Dynamics Information Technology Company (GDIT, Inc.)
Past Chair, NCPeds Committee on Child Abuse and Neglect

**Jane Meschan Foy, MD, FAAP**
(see *Acknowledgements: NCPeds Steering Committee*)

**Gregory K. Griggs, MPA, CAE**
Executive Vice President and CEO, NC Academy of Family Physicians

**Emily A. Hannon, MD, IBCLC, FAAP**
Pediatrician and Owner, Western Wake Pediatrics, Cary, NC
Member, Executive Committee, AAP Section on Breastfeeding
Co-Coordinator for North Carolina, AAP Chapter Breastfeeding

**R. M. "Mac" Herring, Jr., MD, FAAP**
Pediatrician, Clinton Medical Clinic, Clinton, NC (Retired 2014)
Governor's Council on Educational Services for Exceptional Children (1978-86), Chairman (1982-86)
Clinton City Schools Board of Education (1982-90)
Medical Advisory Committee for Sampson County Head Start (1975-95)
Member, Department of Public Instruction/Department of Human Resources Committee on
    Health Assessment of Kindergarten Children (1983)
NC State Health Education Advisory Committee (1989-95)
Child Health Committee, NC State Medical Society (1980-97), Chairman (1992-97)

**Emily Horney, MHA, RDH**
Early Childhood Oral Health Coordinator, Division of Public Health, Oral Health Section,
    NC Department of Health and Human Services

**David Horowitz, MD, FAAP**
Pediatrician, Triangle Pediatrics, Cary, NC
Past Member, NC Council on Developmental Disabilities
Founding Member, Wake County Child Fatality Task Force and Wake County Child Protection Team
Past Chair, NCPeds Mental Health Committee
Executive Committee Member, AAP Section on Ambulatory Practice Management

**William C. (Bill) Hubbard, MD, FAAP**
Pediatrician, Founder of Raleigh Pediatric Associates, Raleigh NC
Clinical Professor, University of North Carolina Department of Pediatrics
Member, multiple local boards focused on children's welfare
Past President, NC Peds

**Elizabeth Hudgins, MPP**
Executive Director, NCPeds (2014 to present)

**Olson Huff, MD, FAAP**
(see *Acknowledgements: NCPeds Steering Committee*)

**Susan H. Huffman, CMPE**
Practice Administrator, Unifour Pediatrics, Hickory, NC
Past Chair, NCPeds Practice Managers Section
Past Member, NCPeds Board of Directors

**Michelle Hughes, MA, MSW**
Owner, Michelle Hughes Consulting
Former Executive Director of NC Child (2014-2022)

**James Baxter Hunt Jr., JD**
Politician and Retired Attorney
27th Lieutenant Governor of North Carolina (1973-77)
69th and 71st Governor of North Carolina (1977-85, 1993-2001)

**Henry Jones Jr., JD**
Attorney and Partner, Jordan Price Wall Gray Jones & Carlton, PLLC, Raleigh, NC
Past Lobbyist for NCPeds

**Martha Ann Keels, DDS, PhD**
Duke Street Pediatric Dentistry
Associate Consulting Professor in Surgery, Duke University
Adjunct Associate Professor in Pediatrics, Duke University
Adjunct Professor in Pediatric Dentistry, Adams University of North Carolina School of Dentistry
Diplomate, American Board of Pediatric Dentistry
Fellow, American Academy of Pediatric Dentistry, American College of Dentists,
    International College of Dentists, Pierre Fauchard Academy
Chair, AAP Section on Oral Health (2004-10)

**Kelly Kimple, MD, MPH, FAAP**
Senior Medical Director for Health Promotion and NC Title V Maternal & Child Director
Division of Public Health, NC Department of Health and Human Services

**Rebecca King, DDS, MPH**
State Dental Director, Section Chief, Oral Health Section
NC Department of Health and Human Services (Retired 2014)

**Colleen Kraft, MD, MBA, FAAP**
Professor of Pediatrics, Keck School of Medicine/University of Southern California
and Children's Hospital Los Angeles
Past AAP President (2018)

**Mike Lawless, MD, FAAP**
Professor of Pediatrics, Wake Forest University School of Medicine (Retired)
Former Division Chief, General Pediatrics and Adolescent Medicine
Former Chair, NCPeds Transportation Safety Committee

**William W. Lawrence, Jr., MD, FAAP**
Chief Medical Officer, Carolina Complete Health, Charlotte, NC
Past Board Member, NCPeds
Past Medical Director and Acting Agency Director, NC Medicaid
Past Board Member, NC Medical Journal

**Matthew R. Ledoux, MD, FAAP**
Interim Chair, Department of Pediatrics, Brody School of Medicine, East Carolina University
Pediatrician-in-Chief, Maynard Children's Hospital at ECU Health Medical Center

**Gerri L. Mattson, MD, MSPH, FAAP**
Senior Medical Director, Division of Child and Family Well-Being,
NC Department of Health and Human Services
Past Member: NCPeds Board Relations Committee, Fostering Health NC
Advisory Committee, and Transition Age Youth Work Group
Member, Executive Board, AAP Council on Community Pediatrics

**Allison Shivers McBride, MD, FAAP**
Associate Professor of Pediatrics and Emergency Medicine
Executive Vice Chair, Department of Pediatrics
Wake Forest University School of Medicine

**John Meidl**
Events and Membership Manager, NCPeds (2014-15)
Veteran US Air Force, Graduate of Campbell University, Buies Creek, NC

**David Millsaps, MD, FAAP**
Lead Pediatrician, Unifour Pediatrics PA, Hickory, NC

**Susan Mims, MD, MPH, FAAP**
President and CEO, Dogwood Health Trust
Past Chair, Department of Community and Public Health, UNC Health Sciences,
Mountain Area Health Education Center
Past Vice President for Children's Services, Chief of Pediatrics, Vice Chief of Staff,
Mission Health System
Past President, NCPeds

**Peter J. Morris, MD, MPH, MDIV, FAAP, FACPM**
Executive Director, Urban Ministries of Wake County
Practitioner of Pediatrics, Public Health, Preventive Medicine, Hospital Medicine
Former Medical Director, Wake County Human Services Agency
Past President, NCPeds

**Dale A. Newton, MD, FAAP**
Professor Emeritus of Pediatrics, Brody School of Medicine, East Carolina University
Former Clinical Professor of Medicine, Senior Vice Chair of Pediatrics, East Carolina University
Former Medical Director, Department of Physician Assistant Studies, East Carolina University
Former Director, Combined Internal Medicine-Pediatrics Residency Program,
    East Carolina University
Formerly in private practice, Tarboro, NC

**Kathryn P. Nichol, MD, MS, FAAP**
Retired Pediatrician and WI Resident
Past Member, AAP Board of Directors

**H. Stacy Nicholson, MD, MPH, FAAP**
Sara H. and Howard C. Bissell Endowed Chair, Chair of Pediatrics and President,
    Atrium Health Levine Children's Hospital, Charlotte, NC
Charlotte Campus Chair of Pediatrics, Wake Forest University School of Medicine
Former Faculty, Children's National Hospital, Washington, DC
Former Chair, Pediatrics, Oregon Health & Science University
Former Physician-in-Chief, Phoenix Children's Hospital
Former Chair, Board of Directors, American Board of Pediatrics (2021)

**Lourdes Pereda, MD, FAAP**
Pediatrician, Kidz Pediatrics, Angier, NC
NCPeds Board of Directors
Member, Peruvian American Medical Society

**J. Duncan Phillips, MD, FACS, FAAP**
Surgeon-in-Chief, WakeMed Children's Hospital
Associate Professor of Surgery, UNC Chapel Hill School of Medicine
Past Chair, NCPeds Subspecialty Committee

**William R. Purcell, MD, FAAP**
The Purcell Clinic, Laurinburg, NC
Captain, US Army Medical Corps 57th Field Hospital, Toul, France (1957-59)
Member of Laurinburg City Council (1982-87)
Mayor of Laurinburg (1987-97)
NC State Senator (1997-2013)

**Ann M. Reed, MD**
Samuel L. Katz Distinguished Professor and Chair, Department of Pediatrics
Pediatrician-in-Chief, Duke University
Clinician-Investigator in Rheumatology and Immunology

**Kenneth B. Roberts, MD, FAAP**
Professor Emeritus of Pediatrics, University of North Carolina School of Medicine
Former Director, Pediatric Teaching Program, Moses Cone Hospital, Greensboro, NC
First Chair, NCPeds Committee on Education
Past President, Association of Pediatric Program Directors
Past President, Ambulatory Pediatric Association
Former Member, Board of Directors, American Board of Pediatrics
AAP Joseph W. St. Geme Jr. Leadership Award
First Recipient, Pediatric Hospital Medicine Lifetime Achievement Award

**Beth Rowe-West, RN, BSN**
NC Immunization Branch, DHHS
Former Public Health Nurse, Davidson County Health Department
Consultant for National Non-Profit Immunization Organizations
Past Member, NCPeds Board of Directors

**R. Gary Rozier, DDS, MPH**
Professor Emeritus, Health Policy and Management, Gillings School of Global Public Health
University of North Carolina, Chapel Hill, NC

**John W. Rusher, MD, JD, FAAP**
Pediatrician and Partner, Raleigh Pediatric Associates, Raleigh & Garner, NC
Past President, NCPeds
Past Chair, NCPeds Legislative Committee
Former Member, AAP Committee on State Government Affairs
Former Member, AAP Committee on Medical Liability and Risk Management
Former Board Member and Past President, NC Medical Board

**Francis Rushton, MD, FAAP**
Pediatrician, Beaufort Pediatrics, Beaufort, SC
Clinical Professor of Pediatrics, University of South Carolina
Medical Director, South Carolina QTIP (Statewide Ambulatory QI Collaborative)
Former Member, AAP Board of Directors

**Scott St. Clair, MD, FAAP**
Pediatrician, Blue Ridge Pediatrics and Adolescent Medicine, Boone, NC
Past President, NCPeds
Past Co-Chair, NCPeds Career Days for Residents

**Robert (Bob) P. Schwartz, MD, FAAP**
(see *Acknowledgements: NCPeds Steering Committee*)

**Sara H. Sinal, MD, FAAP**
Professor Emerita of Pediatrics, Wake Forest School of Medicine
Longstanding Member, NC Committee on Child Abuse and Neglect

**Steve Shore, MSW**
(see *Acknowledgements: NCPeds Steering Committee*)

**David (Dave) T. Tayloe Jr., MD, FAAP**
(see *Acknowledgements: NCPeds Steering Committee*)

**Elizabeth Cuervo "Betsey" Tilson, MD, MPH, FAAP**
NC State Health Director and Chief Medical Officer, NC Department of Health and Human Services
Former Medical Director, Community Care of Wake county and Johnston county
Former Chief Network Medical Director, Community Care of North Carolina
Former Assistant Consulting Professor and Cancer Control Specialist, Duke University
Former Primary Care Pediatrician

**Jon B. Tingelstad, MD, FAAP (Deceased 2023)**
Professor Emeritus of Pediatrics, East Carolina University School of Medicine
Former Chair, Department of Pediatrics, East Carolina University School of Medicine
Former Associate Professor of Pediatrics, Medical College of Virginia

**Emily B. Vander Schaff, MD, MPH, FAAP**
Co-Chair, NCPeds Policy Committee
Member, AAP Community Action to Child Health (CATCH) Executive Committee
AAP District IV CATCH Facilitator

**Tom Vitaglione, MPH**
Child/Family Advocate, NC Child
Former Head, Child Health, Division of Public Health,
    NC Department of Health and Human Services
Senior Fellow, NC Child

**Tork Wade, MPH**
Special Assistant to the President, Community Care of NC
Past Director, NC Office of Rural Health and Community Care of NC

**Dave Williams, MD, FAAP**
Pediatrician, Thomasville/Archdale Pediatrics
Past Chair, NCPeds Membership Committee
Past President, NCPeds
Past District VII Vice-Chair, AAP

**Chuck Willson, MD, FAAP**
Clinical Professor of Pediatrics, Brody School of Medicine, East Carolina University
Past President, NCPeds
Past President, NC Medical Society

**Charlene Wong, MD, MSHP**
Assistant Secretary for Children and Families, NC Department of Health and Human Services
Pediatrics and Public Policy, Duke University School of Medicine
Executive Director, North Carolina Integrated Care for Kids, Duke-Margolis Center for Health Policy